Lubov Grigorenko

Legalizing euthanasia. The illusion of safety

Lubov Grigorenko

Legalizing euthanasia. The illusion of safety

Monograph

ScienciaScripts

Imprint

Any brand names and product names mentioned in this book are subject to trademark, brand or patent protection and are trademarks or registered trademarks of their respective holders. The use of brand names, product names, common names, trade names, product descriptions etc. even without a particular marking in this work is in no way to be construed to mean that such names may be regarded as unrestricted in respect of trademark and brand protection legislation and could thus be used by anyone.

Cover image: www.ingimage.com

This book is a translation from the original published under ISBN 978-3-659-87451-2.

Publisher:
Sciencia Scripts
is a trademark of
Dodo Books Indian Ocean Ltd. and OmniScriptum S.R.L publishing group

120 High Road, East Finchley, London, N2 9ED, United Kingdom
Str. Armeneasca 28/1, office 1, Chisinau MD-2012, Republic of Moldova, Europe
Managing Directors: Ieva Konstantinova, Victoria Ursu
info@omniscriptum.com

Printed at: see last page
ISBN: 978-620-3-28849-0

LUBOV VIKTOROVNA GRIGORENKO
MONOGRAPHY.
LEGALIZING EUTHANASIA IS AN ILLUSION OF SAFETY.
MODERN DISEASES OF CIVILIZATION

The monograph analyzes the medical problem of euthanasia, legalized in civilized countries of the world, one of its legal forms of implementation - assisted suicide with medical assistance; presents medical and social aspects of the problem of euthanasia, describes known from literature sources clinical cases of patients' return after clinical death; describes, studied according to foreign literature sources, clinical features of the course of the most dangerous and practically incurable for a human being modern diseases of civilized countries; describes the clinical features of the course of the most dangerous and practically incurable for a human being modern diseases of civilized countries.

Reviewer s:

Buryak L.I. - Doctor of Medical Sciences, Professor of the Department of Hygiene and Ecology "DMA MZU", Academician of the Academy of Sciences of Ukraine, scientific director of the laboratory H-BTK "Hygienist" and research laboratory H-BTK "Expertise". Author of more than 300 scientific works: including 2 monographs; 5 inventions; 35 proposals.

Shchudro S.A. - Doctor of Medical Sciences, Associate Professor of the Department of Hygiene and Ecology "DMA MZU". Author of more than 80 scientific publications, including about 60 journal articles, 11 normative and methodological documents, 3 monographs and 3 textbooks.

CONTENTS.

" There are two true tragedies in this world. One is the lack of what one would like to possess, the other is that one gets exactly what one would like to have"

Oscar Wilde

INTRODUCTION

Before I move on to examine the philosophical problem of euthanasia from the perspective of philosophers, sociologists, medical, legal and many other specialists, I will quote from the autobiography of Johnny Erekson, who was paralyzed in an accident and about her struggle with her circumstances .

" If you think about it: what is a minute? Part of time. An hour consists of sixty minutes, a day of 1440 minutes. And at the age of seventeen, over nine million minutes have already been lived.

"I looked at the ventilation grate, at the cracked ceiling whitewash. I tried to turn my head to see what was around me, but I couldn't move. The stabbing pain on both sides of my head restricted my movement. Suddenly I imagined it was because of the holes in my skull. When I got up and looked over, I saw large metal tongs attached to some kind of apparatus. I felt as if my head had been ripped off. It took a lot of strength - both bodily and mental - to start to perceive the world around me again.

"I was constantly haunted by drug-induced visions. I often dreamed that I was in some unusual arena with my friend Jes Leverton. We're awaiting trial. In this vision I would suddenly find myself standing in front of a figure in flowing robes, and I knew it was the Apostle. He did not say a word, and it was clear to me that I was to be judged. Suddenly he drew a sharp sword and cut off my head with it. This vision haunted me constantly.

"Tom was a young man who also had a diving accident. The funny thing is that although I knew Tom had broken his spine, it never occurred to me that the same thing had actually happened to me. No one told me that. Tom couldn't breathe on his own. I found this out when I asked my sister what that peculiar noise meant. She explained to me that it was Tom's breathing apparatus. At night, when the fever was slightly subsiding, I could hear the moans of others. That's when I would listen to the continuous noise of Tom's breathing apparatus. Since I couldn't turn and look at him, the noise had a calming effect on me. I felt like I was invisibly connected to him. Later that night, the breathing apparatus suddenly subsided. The silence seemed as loud as an explosion. Panic gripped me, I choked as I wanted to scream for help.... The noise reached our room, I heard a sigh of relief and someone said: "I have a device, please make room for it". But then, to my horror, I heard a cold objection: "Leave it, it's too late. He's dead."

"The horror that seized me did not go away the next day. I grieved for a man I did not know, and then I began to reflect on my own situation. True, I didn't need a machine to breathe. But

I depended on IVs to give my body nourishment, depended on catheters to remove waste products from my body. What happens if one of them fails? What if the forceps at my head weakened? What if. and I was overcome with a thousand fears."

"Two days later a man was admitted with an injury similar to mine. He was put on the same bed under an oxygen hood. When I looked to the side, I saw what the bed actually looked like. I couldn't see my own, I only understood what was happening when I was turned: two hours face up, two hours face down. It seemed to me that we were like bulls being turned on a spit. Whenever I was turned, I was terrified. The new patient was as afraid as I was. When the orderlies wanted to turn him one day, he exclaimed with despair: "No, please don't turn me! The last time you turned me, I couldn't breathe. Please don't turn me!"

- Honey, but it's okay. Nothing's gonna happen to you. We're gonna have to turn you around. You ready, Mike? When I say "three," we're gonna go, "one, two, three!"

- No! Please, no! I can't breathe! I'm sure I'm gonna pass out!

- It's all right. Don't worry! They secured the oxygen hood and left.

As I heard the man's heavy breathing, I prayed that the two hours would pass quickly, for his sake and for my own. Suddenly the breathing was interrupted. The frantic rush began again, with the sisters and aides doing what they could. But it was too late. Another had died. Hot tears rolled down my cheeks. I was again overcome by the fear and despair that had been my constant companions during those first days. With increasing horror, I became more and more aware that the intensive care unit was a room of death. I felt that my own life was hanging by a thread and could not understand how I was still alive. Shortly afterwards, as I was being turned over, I also lost consciousness and stopped breathing. However, within minutes brought me back to life."

"I knew I was on my deathbed, had a premonition that I was going to die like Tom, like that other man. They had injuries similar to mine. So I thought the doctors were considering the possibility of my death. They're just afraid to tell me."

"I lay in the semi-darkness of the ward. I should have been happy that the operation had been successful, that I was recovering. I was in a solitary ward. But I still couldn't rejoice. I was overcome with sadness and despair. For the first time since the accident, I prayed to die.

- Jackie! -I was getting angry. -Get me a mirror and immediately...

"The face in the mirror barely resembled a human face. When I looked at my reflection, I saw dark circles surrounding my eyes, which were glassy in deep hollows. I had lost weight from

67kg to 44kg and looked like a yellowish skinned ghost. The shaved head emphasized my skeleton-like appearance even more. As I mouthed the words, I saw my teeth. They were covered in black plaque from various medications. From that moment on, I was close to suicide.

- Jackie, you have to help me. They're only keeping me alive. But it's not fair. I'm going to die anyway. Why won't they just let me die? Jackie, please, you have to help me! I begged her.

- But what about it, Joni?

- I don't know. Give me something, you know, give me lots of pills.

- Are you saying I should kill you?" Jackie asked, her eyes wide.

- Yeah, I guess. No, you couldn't have killed me. You could just help me die a little sooner. Think, please, I'm almost dead already. Wouldn't you help me reduce my suffering? If I could move, I'd do it myself!

I became embittered and desperate.

-I beg you, slit my wrists, I can't feel anything. It won't hurt. But then I'll die, Jackie. Please do something!"

"I thought through many plans on how to carry out my decision. Taking the extra pills would be the easiest, but the sisters could find out quickly and start pumping her stomach. Sure, Jackie could slit her wrists. I could hide my hands under the sheet, but it still wouldn't work. The only thing left was to hope for some hospital accident that would kill me.

"Life here is like living in an ivory tower. Everyone here is in more or less the same position. If you spend enough time confined to a chair, then you can go home. And it's much easier to live with people in the same position as you. But when you leave the asylum, it's really hard. People on the outside think that if your legs are paralyzed, there must be something wrong with your head. They treat you like an idiot. That's why everyone is eager to come back here, mentally comparing their bodily and mental injuries with others.

I believe that several factors contribute to suicidal thoughts, as exemplified by the critically ill Joni: Intolerable pain as a result of an injury, or surgery (passage 2), constant nightmares, hallucinations and fears (passages 3, 4, 5), deaths of patients with similar diagnoses that occur in front of such people (passages 4, 5) and the realization that medical personnel do not always provide timely help, the realization of one's helplessness and inferiority as a result of a physical ailment, realization that you exist at the level of fulfilling basic physiological needs, inadequate social perception of such "cripples" (excerpts 4, 7), for women, first of all, the change of their appearance plays a role, maybe even more than the pain from the trauma (excerpt 7). Joni displays a kind of "psychological connection" to people who, like herself, are unable to fend for themselves. She deeply experiences the death of each of them and prepares for her own. In this connection, she gradually develops a special worldview: she realizes that life has no meaning: "There is no higher meaning to life. Life is transient, it is conditioned by chance. Labor, family, friendship - stages on the way to death. You exist only for a short time.

In addition, as I think from the example of the description, the fact that there were two deaths is evident: the medical staff, represented by the orderlies, did not listen at all to the pleas of the patient connected to the oxygen hood not to turn him over, and in a few minutes death had already occurred (excerpt 5). Nevertheless, no one paid attention to this case. And besides, this is the second case of a patient's death due to inattention on the part of the nursing staff. And the first patient, Tom? Can we consider that he died from untimely delivery of the breathing apparatus (excerpt 4) and consider the actions of the medical staff as a consequence of negligence? And how many other patients are there like him? [3].

CHAPTER 1
DIFFERENCES BETWEEN INTENTION AND FORESIGHT IN
MEDICAL TERMINATION DECISIONS
LIFE

1.1. ***Traditional distinctions between acts and omissions causing or not causing death and intentions/anticipation of death cannot serve to distinguish consistently between permissible and impermissible decisions to end life***

In many countries, it is appalling that doctors are engaged in activities that result in the foreseeable death of patients. Under certain circumstances, they may refuse life-sustaining treatment or administer lethal doses of pain and symptom-relieving drugs, fully aware of the "***double effect***" of these doses. However, in most countries, physicians are not permitted to intentionally end the lives of their patients by prescribing or administering non-therapeutic lethal drugs, i.e. euthanasia.

Prior to the Northern Territory of Australia's Rights of the Terminally Ill Act (1995), the Netherlands was the only country in the world where doctors could explicitly and deliberately end the life of terminally ill patients at the patient's own request, although euthanasia and physician-assisted suicide remain illegal in that country, the Dutch parliament recognized that doctors practicing it should not be prosecuted if they followed certain rules.

Death is no longer the natural event it once was. On the contrary, most patients die in a hospital setting, as a result of a medical decision to end life. Almost 40% of all deaths (and 54% of all non-acute deaths) are the result of a medical decision to end life: this can be by withholding life-sustaining treatment, administering symptomatic and potentially life-shortening pain medication, and euthanasia.

In all of these cases, doctors deliberately carry out decisions knowing or believing that it will lead to the death of their patients. This means that the relevant issue is not whether or not doctors should be allowed to end the lives of their patients, but when they are allowed to do so.

Consider the following cases:

Mr. Angels, Dr. Adams' patient, is dying of a progressive debilitating disease. He is almost completely paralyzed and needs an "artificial lung" machine to keep him alive. He is suffering greatly and wants to die. He asks the doctor to disconnect the machine. Dr. Adams agrees and Mr. Angels dies three hours later from respiratory failure.

Mr. Brown, Dr. Bernard's patient, is dying of the same disease as Mr. Angels. He also needs an "artificial lung" machine to keep him alive and wants to die. He asks Dr. Bernard to give him an injection of a lethal agent. Dr. Bernard agrees and gives him an injection of potassium chloride. Mr. Brown dies a few minutes later.

Mr. Charles, Dr. Clemens' patient, is suffering from throat cancer that threatens him with death by suffocation. Suffering greatly, he asks Dr. Clemens to end his life. She explains to him that this is impossible, but that she will gradually increase the dosage of painkillers and symptom relieving medications. She says that after a day or two, the doses will be such that Mr. Charles will die as a result of her efforts to relieve his suffering. Dr. Clemens starts the medication and 18 hours later Mr. Charles dies.

Mr. David, Dr. Daisy's patient, is in literally the same position as Mr. Charles. At the patient's request to end his life, Dr. Daisy administers a lethal dose of potassium chloride, and within minutes the patient dies.

In many countries, what Drs. Adams and Clemens did is legal. At the same time, what Drs. Bernard and Daisy did is illegal. Is that right? This issue was addressed in a recent decision by the U.S. Court of Appeals for the Ninth Circuit, Compassion for the Dying v. State of Washington. In his carefully reasoned opinion, supported by a majority of eight to three, Judge Reinhardt recorded that in order for the state to reasonably support a ban on euthanasia, it would be necessary to identify a substantial difference between euthanasia and "conduct ... that the state explicitly recognizes." He argued that in this case it is not sufficient to explain the distinction between acting and refraining from acting. In many cases, refusers of treatment unquestionably commit acts that result in the foreseeable death of their patients.

The case is not helped by even considering the concept of causation. A physician who discontinues treatment causes death, with the same certainty if he were to administer a lethal injection. While we might say that it is the disease that will cause death, he argued that this is not the case when the physician applies a life-shortening palliative treatment. In that case, it is the physician, not the disease, that causes death. Judge Reinhard concluded that in all of these cases, "there is no doubt that the physician implies that as a result of his action the patient will die."

This is a groundbreaking opinion, at odds with the traditional moral principle of "*double jeopardy*" and with the prevailing view of the law. If we accept the view of this court, not only Drs. Bernard and Daisy, but also Drs. Adams and Clemens intended to cause the death of their patients. However, under the prevailing views of the law, only Drs. Bernard and Daisy committed unlawful acts, while Drs. Adams and Clemens would be considered to have adhered to good medical practices.

Should we stick to the conventional wisdom? In my opinion, no. There is good reason to agree with Judge Reinhardt's conclusion that the law should cease to distinguish between permissible and impermissible end-of-life decisions on the basis of concepts such as *acting-abstaining from acting, causing-not causing death, and most importantly, intending-not intending to cause death.*

1.2. *Laws that prohibit doctors from practicing euthanasia, are discriminatory and unfair*

The main argument is that the conventional view unfairly discriminates against patients who have reached the end of their lives, are suffering and want to die. This issue was raised in another court case of great importance in the United States: Timothy E. Quill et al. v. State of New York. Based on the legal permissibility for doctors to discontinue treatment, Quill argued:

" *Removal of a life support system that results in the death of the patient requires the direct involvement of a physician. When such patients are in a sane state, they consciously choose death as a preferable solution to living under the circumstances in which they are forced to live. However, some dying patients in agony who cannot be relieved of their suffering but who are not dependent on life-sustaining treatment have no such choice under existing legal restrictions. It is unjust and arbitrary and inhumane to deprive some dying patients of such an important choice because of such arbitrary conditions of their lives that determine whether they depend on life-support systems that can be stopped.*"

The Court of Appeals agreed and enjoined medically assisted suicide on the grounds that it discriminates against patients who are "unlucky" because they do not require a life support system that they can refuse.

1.3. *Flexibility and the possibility of ambiguous interpretation of the decision to termination of life*

This argument seems very convincing. Can it be argued that weakening the ban on euthanasia could have worse consequences? Probably not. In addition to the fact that people are treated unfairly, there is no publicity or legal protection in the current situation.

The problem lies in the concept of *intention (envisioning).*

The conventional wisdom is that doctors do not foresee all foreseeable consequences of their actions. This encourages extreme flexibility and arbitrary interpretation of end-of-life decisions. Doctors who, for whatever reason, do not wish to practice "euthanasia" have other means to achieve the same result. Instead of using potassium chloride, Drs. Bernard and Daisy could, for example, use common therapeutic drugs to hasten the deaths of their patients, and in doing so, their actions would move from criminal homicide to "good medical practice".

Of course, patients could die within hours or days rather than within minutes, but that has nothing to do with the doctors' intentions.

Moreover, if doctors who perform these slower types of lethal acts are thought to have no intention of ending their patients' lives, can it be said that those who use faster means have such intentions?

This issue was raised at the trial of Dr. Jack Kevorkian, who was accused of assisting in ending the lives of two terminally ill individuals, but was acquitted by a jury. Under Michigan law, "a person is not guilty of criminal assisted suicide if that person administered medications and procedures with the intent to relieve pain and discomfort rather than cause death," even if such treatment "may hasten or increase the risk of death." Dr. Kevorkian's claim that he did not intend for his patients to die is unconvincing. This case speaks to the possibility of different interpretations of end-of-life decisions, as well as the fact that we are dealing with subjective (as well as objective) notions of intent. No one thinks that doctors envision all foreseeable and likely "only" consequences of their life-shortening actions or refusal to act.

If intent is understood in a broad "objective" sense, then death resulting from any deliberate medical decision to end life (so that death is not accidental or unintentional) should be considered an intended consequence. Since this is not the generally accepted view, it follows that existing bylaws and laws are based on a subjective notion of intent [!Griffith: The Regulation of Ethanasia]. This means that often only the physician himself can say whether he foresaw the death of the patient or merely anticipated it as an inevitable consequence of what he did.

" *This means that regulating and controlling end-of-life decisions will be very difficult, if not impossible. Even if the distinctions between directly intended and merely foreseen consequences have some meaning in abstract philosophical or theological discussions, they mean little at the patient's bedside.*"

As John Griffith writes: "*The medical decisions involved follow so closely one after the other, and the whole decision-making process is so situation-specific, that identifying when a doctor's intention has changed from 'pain relief' to 'death' (with the consequence that very different legal rules are involved) is entirely arbitrary. Doctors can hardly be blamed for framing medical end-of-life decisions in the way that is most convenient for them".*

That is, the conventional view does not encourage honesty and openness in the doctor-patient relationship, nor does it encourage the consent of the patient. If the patient requests the use of euthanasia and the physician consents, the latter (controversially) participates in the deliberate termination of life, whether by administering therapeutic or non-therapeutic means or by terminating life support. If this issue is not raised and the patient's consent is not asked, it is much easier to describe medical termination of life decisions simply as representing "good medical practice."

If we accept the consent of the patient in medical end-of-life decisions as the central law-forming aspect of such actions, then we have to take into account the consequences of this. A large-scale study in the Netherlands shows that even in a country where euthanasia can be openly practiced, the majority of patients die as a consequence of non-euthanasia type decisions and very many die without giving their consent [1, 2, 3, 5].There is reason to believe that, as far as patient consent is concerned, the situation is probably even worse in countries where euthanasia is not permitted.

It follows from all of the above that we should stop asking whether a physician "intends" to cause death or whether he or she simply "allows" it to happen. These distinctions may be morally relevant in the context of any moral or religious views, but they are not an adequate basis for a societal approach to end-of-life issues. What is needed is a unified regulatory framework for all medical end-of-life decisions, the basis of which rests not on subjective notions of intention but on procedural safeguards such as the patient's consent [6].

CHAPTER 2
IS EUTHANASIA A MERCY KILLING?

People are known to be afraid of death. Sometimes panic-stricken. Realizing its inevitability, one cannot but agree with the ancient philosopher Seneca, who said: "Death is the law, not the punishment.

Euthanasia means "easy death" in Greek. Euthanasia is the right of a person to die, to kill in the name of compassion. There is, as it turns out, such a right. And this is one of the peculiarities of the dialectic of life.

One point of view prevails in our country: no euthanasia, medicine exists only to help the sick and prevent diseases, not to kill people. To prove it, I will cite below the results of a sociological study conducted in 1991-1992 by the Finnish Institute of Occupational Health and the Institute of Sociology. The Finnish Institute of Occupational Health and the Institute of Sociology of the Russian Academy of Sciences on the topic: "Professional and family roles of doctors". Among other things, the respondents were asked several questions in the field of biomedical ethics [1].

The problem of euthanasia dates back to the times of ancient Greece and Rome. The increased interest to it in modern conditions is due to the fact that despite the progress of medicine, mortality in a number of serious diseases is still high.

In the U.S. state of Oregon, under the Death and Dignity Act of 1997, any adult of sound mind who has been certified by several physicians that he or she will not live beyond one month may request a medical facility to provide him or her with a drug to "end his or her suffering and end his or her life in a humane and dignified manner. The physician who prescribes such a drug does not administer it. The patient must take the "medicine" himself.

This does not mean, however, that euthanasia is legal in the United States. In most states in this country, the law provides for serious criminal liability for those who assist another to commit suicide.

Foreign authors draw attention to the fact that the vast majority of patients with terminal diseases (primarily cancer) who wish to leave life are in a state of depression, obsessive suicidal ideation. Therefore, it is important to realize that the idea of suicide is not the same as a patient's request for euthanasia.

It is often suggested in the literature that inadequate treatment in the Netherlands may be a reason for requesting euthanasia. It is difficult to agree with this, but it is certainly likely that the suffering of the dying patient goes far beyond physical pain. Other factors such as loss of mobility, loss of activity, combined with a growing sense of hopelessness and dependence on others can cause severe distress. Another component of suffering is the loss of self-esteem. Although this is a very subjective component, the patient finds it very important. This is confirmed by research in the Netherlands.

In 1990, patients requested euthanasia for the following reasons:

- *loss of self-esteem-57%,*

- *pain-46%,*

- *undignified dying-46%,*

- *dependence on others-33%,*

- *fatigue with life-23%.*

In only 10 out of 187 cases was pain cited as the sole cause. The results of these studies echo the findings of other studies, also conducted in the Netherlands, according to which pain was the most important reason in only 5% of cases. It turned out that patients accustomed to tolerating pain were less eager to be euthanized than those suffering from depression. The Dutch example shows that the main reasons for requests for euthanasia are loss of self-esteem and the unworthy process of dying, which the patient considers completely unacceptable [7]. In 1995, Pope John Paul II delivered one of the strongest condemnations of abortion and euthanasia at the Vatican, saying that legalizing them was equivalent to legalizing crimes that destroy society. "*Politicians and laws opposed to life lead society to degeneration, not only morally, but also demographically and economically,*" he *said.* And although 75% of Italians consider themselves Catholics, abortion was legalized in this country in 1978 and supported in a referendum in 1981 [Gazeta "Zerkalo Nedeli".- 2000.- № 44 (from 11.XI)].

2.1.   Some ethical issues arising in post-Soviet countries

Recently, the press has begun to publish reports by journalists about possible violations of medical ethics by doctors when removing organs from corpses for further transplantation to patients in need. It is enough to familiarize oneself with the content of articles published in newspapers

[Komsomolskaya Pravda.-1991.-13 December; 1992.-20 March; Kommersant.- 1991.-#40 (30 September-6 October); Kuranty.-1992.-#3; Arkh.pat.-1978.-#9.- pp.1121- 1126], where various ethical problems of transplantation, including commercial issues of "organ trade" are considered [Komsomolskaya Pravda.-1992.-March 19; USSR. Ministry of Health. Order 191 of 15.02.85; Kommersant.-1991.-#44].

At the same time, there is an impression that both journalists and resuscitation doctors are not sufficiently aware of the unique condition of the human body, in which brain death occurs while the heart is working.

As it is known, for many centuries human death has been recognized only after cessation of cardiac activity and respiration. Application of resuscitation methods allowed to identify a new state of human organism - brain death, in which there is a development of total necrosis of the brain, brain stem and first cervical segments with a working heart. The most difficult moral and ethical problem arose - to recognize a person dead in case of total necrosis of the brain, but with preserved heart activity and to equate brain death to the death of a human being as a whole. Therefore, in a number of countries the establishment of brain death and, therefore, human death has been elevated to the rank of law. The removal of organs in this state is of particular importance for transplantation, since a working heart provides better functional preservation.

The diagnosis of brain death is universally accepted throughout the world. The term "irreversible brain death" should be categorically rejected and equated with the term "brain death". The term "irreversible brain death" is not a diagnosis, but is used by neurologists to refer to extensive processes in the brain resulting in an absent state, sometimes with respiratory failure but preserved heart function and partial brainstem function. Their morphologic basis is extensive multiple infarcts, brain atrophy, hydrocephalus, inflammatory and degenerative processes. All of them form irreversible syndromes well known in neurological practice: apallic or vegetative state, decortication, decerebration syndromes. The life of such patients can be prolonged for many months and years and depends entirely on care and provision of metabolic functions.

The development of legislation on brain death in our country was initiated in 1984. At that time, the CMEA Permanent Commission for Cooperation in Health Care adopted a protocol on the development of criteria for determining brain death. Then the Ministry of Health of the USSR issued Order No. 191 of February 15, 1985 on the approval of the "Temporary Instruction on Death Constantation" [10] [10], which had a section concerning the diagnosis of brain death with a working heart, the Research Institute of Transplantology of Artificial Organs twice submitted the "Regulations on the procedure for the removal of organs from cadaver donors" (June 1985) and the "Instruction on the procedure for the removal of organs and tissues from cadaver donors" (May 1986). These materials did not provide for the information of relatives and their consent to the removal of organs, as well as the will of the deceased, who could during his lifetime (if he was aware of it) bequeath consent to the removal of organs or, on the contrary, reject it. An attending intensive care physician was allowed to participate in the commission to establish brain death, which could facilitate relatives' expressions of distrust in the diagnosis and other objections. In addition, the commission was given the right to authorize the removal of organs, which is unacceptable because it is independent and its purpose is to establish brain death and notify the relatives.

The draft allowed for transportation of a cadaver donor to a medical institution for organ removal, after which the cadaver would be transported for "pathological and anatomical examination to the medical and preventive institution from which it was brought. Performing an autopsy after the removal of organs is hardly acceptable. Critical remarks regarding the regulation and instructions were made twice by the Research Institute of Neurology in June 1985 and May 1986, but were not taken into account.

The lack of respect for the legality of organ removal has given rise to numerous press articles on the subject and even references to the possibility of commercial transactions. At the 44th (44th)session of the World Health Assembly in 1987-1988 "Guidelines regulating transplantation of human organs" were developed. They present human rights concerning the removal of organs with special care, and also prohibit advertising, commercial transactions and receiving money for the human body and its parts. A law of the Russian Federation "On the Transplantation of Human Tissues and Organs" is currently envisaged. There are serious violations in the draft law, which in the future may lead to conflict situations of moral and ethical importance.

First, there is no concept of brain death itself. Instead, the undefined and controversial term "irreversible brain death" is used, which is not a diagnosis but is often used, as mentioned above, for completely different neurological syndromes. Instead of this vague concept, the diagnosis of "brain death" is used worldwide.

Secondly, human rights must be respected impeccably, both during life and after death. For this purpose, awareness of existing legislation on the removal of organs from a corpse is of paramount importance. Only on the basis of informed consent, which is universally accepted as mandatory, can this procedure be carried out.

Human rights are grossly violated in the submitted draft:

"... the *removal of organs from a corpse is allowed provided that the person in question did not object to it during his or her lifetime or if the relatives of the deceased person have not expressed their unwillingness to have his or her body organs and tissues removed for transplantation after death"*. Such "consent" can hardly be called consent, since the deceased during his lifetime may not have been aware of how his body would be treated after death. The relatives of the deceased cannot claim that the deceased was unwilling to have his organs removed during his lifetime, as neither the deceased nor the relatives themselves may be unaware, without special knowledge, of the legislation on the removal of organs from a corpse. Therefore, the first guiding principle states that organ removal is only possible "*if all the types of approvals required by law have been achieved"*. Before the approval of the Law of the Russian Federation "On Transplantation of Human Tissues and Organs", it is necessary to adopt a separate law on brain death, which will ensure compliance with all criteria for establishing brain death, as is done in many countries of the world. The law will contribute to observance of the order of recognizing a person as dead at working heart. This condition is not even mentioned in the draft Act. The Brain Death Act is linked to the protection of human rights and the creation of optimal conditions for organ transplantation [9].

Is it possible to consider the desire of dying patients to die with dignity in such conditions, when the acts of medical workers have legal grounds, and are conditioned to a greater extent by commercial interest. Or maybe the lives of people in need of organ transplants are worth such sacrifices? Then why don't patients who ask doctors to medically end their lives bequeath consent for the removal of their organs to save someone else's life. Perhaps many problems, in my opinion, would be solved. And in such a case we could really talk about mercy, both on the part of the hopeless patients themselves and on the part of medical workers.

2.2. What doctors think about euthanasia

The magazine "Doctor" [4] published an article by L. Durnov "Euthanasia - easy death?" [4] an article by L. Durnov "Euthanasia - an easy death?" was published. In response to this publication there were a lot of comments, both supporters and opponents of euthanasia [7, 8]. The most memorable for me was F. Chumakov's review, and I will quote: *"I have seen many deaths. In most cases it is hard to die. There is a well-known proverb:* **Two deaths cannot happen, but one cannot be avoided**. *By resuscitating a hopeless patient, we condemn him to at least two deaths. I can't forget one laryngeal cancer patient. He died of recurrent arterial* *bleeding as a result of extensive necrosis of the soft tissues of the neck, which occurred as a result of an overdose of gamma radiation during radiation therapy.*

During 10 days he was resuscitated three times (the last time without success). Thus, fulfilling our medical duty, we made this sufferer die three times, having won only 10 days from death. But how he spent those days!"

"It seems to me that some of the 'staunch opponents' of euthanasia, namely those who are not opposed to abortion, are being sanctimonious. In euthanasia, we are fulfilling the will of the patient and helping a hopelessly ill or decrepit old person who can no longer live on earth, an unpromising invalid who does not want to continue in such a position, or a patient suffering from long and intolerable pains. In abortion they kill a child (fetus), which has its whole life ahead of it. It is not known how many geniuses mankind has lost as a result of abortion, what gene pool has been destroyed. So far our laws prohibit euthanasia and allow abortion. How do we understand this?"

Analyzing the statements of a respected person, doctor of medical sciences, regarding the first passage I would like to say: how can one treat a person in such a way that he died as a result of overdose of radiation therapy, and then try to save his life three times, knowing that it is unsuccessful?

As for the second passage, I would like to say to the doctor: God forbid you should ever find yourself such a "decrepit old man" and fall into the hands of the same attending physician who will help you "retire from life".

It seems to me that F. Chumakov judges too harshly, dividing humanity into "geniuses" and all other people. History has already known cases of such a worldview, which led to tragedy (fascist theory of "pure race").

As far as abortion is concerned, it is hard to disagree. The World Medical Association Declaration on Therapeutic Abortion (Oslo, 1970) states:

1.   The primary moral duty of the physician, as articulated in the Declaration of Geneva, is respect for human life: "I shall have the utmost respect for human life from the moment of its conception".

2.   Circumstances that bring the mother's vital interests into conflict with the vital interests of the child create a dilemma: can the pregnancy be intentionally terminated or not?

3.   Different attitudes stem from different attitudes towards the life of the newborn and relate to personal beliefs and conscience that must be respected.

4.   It is not the prerogative of the medical profession to dictate to any state or community the treatment of this subject. It is our responsibility to try to protect our patients and the rights of the physician in the community.

5.   Consequently, where the law allows therapeutic abortion or where legislation on the subject is being debated, and where it is not contrary to the policy of the national medical association and the authorities are prepared to accept the medical profession's position, the following principles should be followed:

•   abortion should only be performed as a therapeutic procedure;

•   The decision to terminate a pregnancy should be made, if possible in writing, by at least two physicians with appropriate professional competence;

•   The procedure is carried out by a suitably qualified doctor in a designated room.

6.   If a physician feels that his or her beliefs do not allow him or her to recommend or perform an abortion, he or she may remove himself or herself by ensuring that the patient receives medical care from a qualified colleague.

7.   This statement, although endorsed by the General Assembly of the World Medical Association, cannot, however, be regarded as binding on those members of the association who do not accept it.

One cannot pass by the article by Lev Abramovich Durnov, director of the Research Institute of Pediatric Oncology and Hematology, which raises the difficult question of the physician's attitude to euthanasia [4].

In its very beginning is this phrase *: "I will not give to any man the deadly remedy asked of me, nor will I show the way for such a design". Hippocrates*

L.A. Durov writes that many seriously ill people have "black" and "light" days, just like healthy people. Constant pain, which can not always be alleviated, the inability to do your favorite work, inclement weather outside the window and the family is bad - what a life it is! But now the pain has receded a little, something can be done, the sun is shining outside the window and my daughter has come - how beautiful life is, despite everything! Very often the request for an "easy death" comes from relatives of the sick. Seeing how unbearably a loved one suffers, and knowing that these are his last days, they ask the doctor to help the dying person to pass away.

In his article, he cites many cases as active euthanasia (where means are used to hasten death): In Michigan, former pathologist Dr. Kevorkian, or "Dr. Death" as he is known, actively euthanized 13 patients; in Australia, the first legal euthanasia of a cancer patient, Dent, was performed; in 1993 the House of Lords allowed Tony Bland, who had been in a coma since 1989 after an injury, to have his IV drip turned off; American doctor Timothy Quill could not refuse a patient with malignant tumor leukemia who asked for a drug that overdoses lead to death ; British rheumatologist Nigel Cox was sentenced to prison for giving potassium cyanide to a patient who had suffered for years from a severe form of rheumatoid arthritis accompanied by excruciating pain; the Tel Aviv District Court granted Mariam Tzadok's request for euthanasia, because she had an incurable form of cancer, and passive euthanasia (when a doctor refuses to do anything to prolong the patient's life).

In addition, he cites cases of euthanasia from fiction: Sidney Sheldon's novel, Rau's book Perversion in Love (the mayor of a French town killed his wife at her request, who had an incurable form of cancer), Christelle and Isabelle Zachert's Meet Me in Paradise, and others. In addition to references to literature, publications in the press and his own cases, of course the doctor did not go along with his patients' requests for euthanasia, Lev Abramovich also refers to laws, to the opinion of the Church, and to the statements of Max Frisch, Epicurus and others.

2.3. Laws

The World Medical Association Declaration of 1981 states: "The patient has the right to die with dignity". This is confirmed by the Russian law on medical care. The state of Michigan has passed a law prohibiting assisted suicide. In the Criminal Code of the RSFSR of 1992, in a note to the article punishing murder, the right to pardon was recognized if the murder was committed out of compassion, at the persistent request of the victim. But this note was withdrawn because too many premeditated murders could be covered by it.

2.4. Church

The Roman Archbishop Clancy wrote: "*The adoration of human life is the cornerstone of civilization. When it disappears, society will disintegrate.*

Another religious figure, Gino Copseti: "*Everyone will be horrified by this outrageous case of euthanasia, which was paid for*".

The Church has always been against suicide, and she is even more so against euthanasia. "*Let us face suicide with the most ardent indignation and we will strike with the word of love anyone who allows himself to treat this grave sin indulgently, lightly and even more approvingly*" - this was said by the priest F. Ornatsky in 1894, when all patients with malignant tumors were dying and there were no modern methods of anesthesia.

2.5. Sayings

Max Frisch: *"It makes no difference whether a person commits suicide or dies a natural death. Voluntary death is the perfect end of life, for all our lives depend on the will of others and only death on our own.*

Prof. Shamov: *"Many times one is convinced that the fight against disease must be fought in any condition of the patient. Not in all cases the doctor is a winner, quite often in terminal conditions we have to swallow the bitter pill of defeat, however, if even only one out of a hundred of such patients comes back to life - and then all the efforts of the doctor are justified".*

Epicurus: *"To Hermachus from Epicurus greetings! When I wrote you this, I was experiencing a happy day, which is together and my last day. I have been haunted by such anguish that nothing, it seems, can be added to its force.*

But to the suffering of the body I counteracted the strength of spirit that came from the recollection of my inventions."

L.Durov's article ends with the following words: What would I ask for myself? Thus, we see two articles and two opposite opinions (F.Chumakov and L.Durov). I think that each of them judges this problem being a materialist and idealist. It is difficult to be a materialistic doctor without spiritual values and soul qualities. It is difficult, first of all, for the patients themselves and their relatives. Sometimes only faith in a "miracle" helps to heal seemingly hopeless patients when they can only hope for a "miracle". I think that a practicing doctor should be both a materialist (in order not to make mistakes based on medical knowledge) and an idealist (in cases when medicine is powerless and one does not want to lose faith in miraculous healing of patients).

2.6. Sociological study of the problem of euthanasia

The respondents were 316 Moscow physicians belonging to different age-gender and professional-medical categories. The question was formulated as follows: "Do you consider euthanasia acceptable?" Four answer options were offered: "Yes, if the patient wishes it", "In exceptional cases", "Under no circumstances", "Never thought about it".

32 respondents (more than 10%) **did not answer** this question at all. This sharply exceeds the number of non-respondents to any other question. Of the four age categories, the highest proportion of non-respondents was in the oldest age groups. As for the medical specialty, the

highest number of non-respondents is among gynecologists and general practitioners (15-20%).

If we summarize the number of non-respondents and those who answered *"Never thought about it (a)",* it turns out that almost half of the respondents did not want to or could not express a definite opinion on this issue. This means that many doctors are not aware of the existence of the problem of euthanasia (or maybe the term itself). It is possible that some part of respondents from these two categories avoided a definite answer because the question seemed to them to be formulated not definitively enough.It is characteristic that a large share of respondents who answered *"I have never thought about it (a)"* belong to older age categories. These data contradict the obvious assumption that doctors with more experience and life practice think more often about life and death issues. Here there is another tendency - higher interest to the problem of euthanasia on the part of young physicians testifies to the change of value attitudes characteristic of professional consciousness of physicians.

More than 40% of those who answered the question and more than 35% of all respondents, contrary to the officially proclaimed legal and ethical norms, believe that euthanasia is permissible in some situations. The same regularity can be traced here: the share of those who chose the first and second answer options *"Yes, if the patient wants it" and "In exceptional cases" is* the highest (49%) among doctors of younger (21-30 years old) age category and decreases in older ones. Perhaps, this is another evidence of the above-mentioned trend, and to some extent the factor of less internalization of professional standards by young specialists is acting.

Of the two positive answers, the reference to the patient's autonomy occurs only in the first case. It is not excluded that in any case the presence or absence of such a desire is not realized by the respondent as a decisive argument. Moreover, the data for the second answer option show that the younger the doctors are, the more inclined they are to allow euthanasia without reference to the patient's opinion.

Do you think euthanasia is acceptable?

Indicator	Yes, if that's what the patient wants	In exceptional cases	Under no circumstances	Never thought about it.	Total
Age (years)					
21-30	7	19	9	17	52
31-40	12	29	14	41	86
41-50	9	16	7	34	66
51-65	14	11	11	30	66
Paul					
Men	20	25	14	38	97
Women	22	50	27	85	159
Specialty					
Psychiatrist	5	10	7	14	36
Pediatrician	3	12	2	25	42
Anesthesiologist	5	11	7	10	26
Surgeon	4	S	9	25	47
Gynecologist	4	6	3	14	27
Therapist	12	13	11	24	60
Neurologist	3	7	2	2	13
Others	6	8	1	10	25
Position					
Professor, Associate Professor	1	1	1	3	6
Chief physician, head of department. and	S	6	5	22	41
Specialist doctor	22	36	20	50	128
Resident	7	17	11	35	70
Others	4	14	3	13	34
Place of work					
RESEARCH INSTITUTE	4	25	15	27	71
Regional Hospital	22	26	18	36	102
Specialized nalizirovan hospital.	2	4	1	10	17
Polyclinic, medical center, etc.	n	16	5	47	79

The indicators for the option ***"Yes, if the patient wants it", on*** the contrary, show that doctors of the oldest age category are most often inclined to be guided by the patient's wish (no significant differences are revealed among other age groups). Apparently, the experience accumulated over many years of direct contact with seriously and hopelessly ill patients and a more concrete understanding of human suffering and death are the reasons for this. Somewhat simplified, we can say that this answer option suggests euthanasia out of compassion, whereas ***"In exceptional cases"*** shifts the emphasis to the practical ineffectiveness of life-sustaining treatment.

As for the evaluation of euthanasia by men and women, the ratio is about 1:2. The proportion of refusals is also similar in both categories.

The data for the response option, *"Never thought about it,"* indicate that women are more likely than men to withhold a definite judgment. However, to the same extent that male physicians are more likely than female physicians to make a definite judgment, they tend to allow euthanasia at the patient's request.

The next factor influencing the attitude to euthanasia is the doctor's specialty. The 4th answer option *"Never thought about it"* was chosen by a relatively small part of anesthesiologists and especially neurologists. The same categories are leading among those who consider euthanasia acceptable, and here neuropathologists are noticeably ahead of all other categories. The fact is that the problem of euthanasia is especially acute in case of irreversible disturbance of brain and central nervous system function. Neurologists more often than others encounter such cases, are more aware of the ineffectiveness of life-sustaining therapy to restore the patient's personality, and therefore are more inclined to consider euthanasia permissible.

Interestingly, doctors of all specialties without exception more often choose the second option *"In exceptional cases"*.

If we exclude pediatricians, because their patients cannot make a competent judgment, the most obvious preference is given to neurologists, anesthesiologists, and psychiatrists, who tend to be guided not only by the subjectively expressed will of the patient, but by an objective assessment of his present and projected condition.

The data on physician's attitude to euthanasia depending on their position are interesting. The most popular category here is specialist physician: it also accounts for the largest share of those who evaded answering (about 15%). At the same time, in the same category, excluding the difficult to interpret category "others", the largest number of respondents chose the 4th option: *"Never thought about it"*.

These respondents, on the one hand, are the closest (along with residents) to the patient, and on the other hand, are more often forced to take the burden of decisions. In general, this category accounted for more than 47% of responses to the two "allowing" euthanasia options. Thus, proximity to the patient's bedside makes the physician more tolerant of euthanasia.

It is also noteworthy that only in the category of chief physicians and heads of departments the number of those who preferred option 4 prevails. Obviously, since such responsible positions are more often occupied by older people, they are more inclined to be guided by the patient's wishes.

The data on the relationship between the place of primary employment and attitude to euthanasia reveal two similar groups: employees of research institutes and doctors of general hospitals, on the one hand, and psychiatric (or other specialized) hospitals, polyclinics and medical stations, on the other. In the first group, there are significantly more of those who have a definite position on euthanasia, both permitting and not permitting it. In the second group there are considerably more of those who preferred the 4th answer option.

This is easy to explain because in outpatient clinics, physicians are less likely to be faced with making life-and-death decisions.

It is noteworthy that among the staff of research institutes there is a very small proportion of those who make the admissibility of euthanasia dependent on the patient's wishes, and, on the contrary, there is a large proportion of those who allow euthanasia in exceptional cases. This is due to the predominance of their research interest over the interest of ensuring the good of the patient. Another factor that may influence this attitude is the complexity of the cases they have to deal with.

On the contrary, for the category of general hospital doctors, the indicators for the first two answer options are quite close, and here, compared to all other categories, the share of those who are inclined to be guided by the patient's wishes is relatively high.

Thus, in conclusion, we can say that more than half of the respondents cannot say anything about euthanasia. Younger doctors show more interest in the problem of euthanasia and are more likely to allow it. At the same time, among those who allow it in general, there are almost twice as few of those who proceed from the patient's wish than those who are guided primarily by objective data on the patient's condition.

There is also a clear trend: the closer doctors are to the "headboard" and the more often they have to deal with patients in critical condition, the more tolerant they are towards euthanasia. Here we meet one of the objective contradictions of scientific and technical progress in the field of biomedicine, when, making it possible to sustain life in situations unimaginable until recently, doctors often prolong the severe suffering of hopelessly ill patients, who do not always consider the actions of doctors towards themselves justified.

The fact that more than 35% of the total number of respondents, contrary to official legal and deontological norms, consider euthanasia to be permissible is particularly eloquent.

Even if not 35 but 95% of all doctors in Russia were in favor of euthanasia, this would not be a sufficient reason for its legalization. The decision can be made only after a broad public discussion, because the meaning of public discussion, as well as the meaning of legal and ethical norms, is to identify and harmonize differently directed interests [10, 11].

As for my opinion on this issue, I believe that euthanasia cannot be legalized. No one can take away the life of a person, especially a hopeless patient. The problem could be solved by the creation of hospices - medical and social institutions for hopeless patients. The doctor is the original savior of life. So how can he take it away? And what about the Hippocratic Oath*: "I will not give anyone a lethal remedy asked of me, nor will I show the way for such an idea"*. In one of the articles [2] one of the arguments of euthanasia supporters is that funds are spent on keeping doomed people alive. It would be better to help the truly needy. And examples are given:

"When they say we should put someone to death to save money, the first thing they name is children with birth defects. Why sick children? Because they can't fight back, they don't yet know their mother by sight, and worst of all, if they are well cared for, they can live a long life and during that long life they consume significant resources. The opportunity to save money on such children is not missed in Germany, where this problem was solved in the mid-30s, or in China: children with congenital defects are kept in specialized orphanages, where they are not cared for, poorly fed. This is the most elementary way of killing - none of these children live more than 2 months."

But if we think this way, maybe we should start saving money on the disabled, the homeless, abandoned children, close nursing homes and shelters for homeless children, or, for example, why not save money on prisoners, because "how many resources they consume"? Why can we "save money" only on defenseless patients and children with birth defects, and not, for example, on criminal offenders: scumbags, maniacs, murderers, rippers? Is it not because hopelessly sick and defenseless children cannot fight back? Their lives are in our hands and they entrust it to us. Often the decision to euthanize is made by tormented relatives or, on the contrary, the sick themselves come to the conclusion that their existence is hopeless because they do not want to be a burden to their relatives. So in relation to whom is euthanasia considered "compassionate mercy"? I, for one, do not see any mercy in euthanasia. Nowadays, medical progress has reached such a level that there is a huge variety of painkillers to relieve pain.

Since one of the large-scale studies conducted in the Netherlands that I described above mentions ***undignified*** dying as a leading cause of the desire to pass away, I turned to the research of Dr. Raymond Moody, who describes the phenomenon of continuing life after the death of the body in his book Life After Life. Will the book I now hold in my hands shed light on understanding what lies behind "dying with dignity"?

CHAPTER 3
IS THERE LIFE AFTER DEATH?

R. Moody's book tells about the real experience of people who were recognized as clinically "dead" and were revived. The testimonies of people who have had such experiences are strikingly similar, down to individual details [6].

In one of the chapters, the author touches on the problem of "the near-death experience of attempted suicide". This kind of experience is unanimously characterized as very painful. As one woman put it:

"*If you leave this world with a suffering soul, your soul will suffer there too*." One man who was distressed by the death of his wife shot himself, "died," but then was revived. He recounts: "*I didn't get to where my wife was. I got to a terrible place ... I saw what a mistake I had made.... I thought: I wish it had not been done by me.*" Others who experienced this unpleasant state said that they felt like they were doomed to be in that position for a long time. They felt it as a punishment for "breaking the rules" by attempting to be prematurely released from life, some kind of "assignment," the fulfillment of a certain life purpose.

People who have experienced this condition have said that suicide is a great misfortune that is accompanied by severe punishment. One person who had a near-death experience during an accident said, "*While I was there, I clearly felt that there were two things that were absolutely forbidden for me, killing myself and killing someone else. If I were to commit suicide, it would mean that I would be throwing God's gift in His face. To kill someone else is to interfere with God's plan for that person.*"

Such sentiments are contained in many testimonies and are found in most ancient theological and moral arguments against suicide. St. Thomas Aquinas argued that life is a divine gift and that it is a divine prerogative, not a human prerogative, to take it.

After reading this, I came to the conclusion that people who ask a doctor for euthanasia want to transfer their "sin of committing suicide" onto the doctor's shoulders. If the doctor agrees to carry out this kind of wish of the patient, his "hands will be covered with the patient's blood" and his death will be on the doctor's conscience.

Those who had experienced "dying" expressed the same idea - that they are no longer afraid of death. However, none of the people interviewed by Moody seeks death or desires it. They all realize that they have certain tasks in this physical life, and certainly reject suicide as a means of returning to the reality in which they have been. It's just that now the state of death doesn't appear to them as something scary, threatening. "*Now I'm not afraid to die. It doesn't mean that death is desirable to me, or that I want to die right now. I don't want to live there now because I believe I should live here. But I am not afraid of death because I know where I will go after I leave this world, since I have been there before."*

The main reason why death ceases to be frightening is that the survivor of such an experience no longer doubts that life does not end with the death of the body. And for such a person it is no longer an abstract possibility, but a fact of his or her own experience.

Some survivors of death describe it as a transition from one state to another, or an exit of consciousness to a higher level of being. One woman who has seen her family come to meet her at the time of "death" compares death to "coming home. Others say, *"Life is like imprisonment. But in this state we simply do not realize what a prison our body is for us. Death is like a release, a getting out of prison. That's probably the best thing I could compare it to.*

In order to understand what attracts survivors to the experience of death, at a certain stage of dying, they do not want to go home:

"I was outside of my physical body and I felt like I had to make a decision.... I realized that I had to decide something: either to move away from here or to go back. On the other hand, it was quite strange, and I still wanted to stay. It was absolutely amazing to realize that I would have to do good on earth. So I thought about it and decided: Yes, I must go back and live."

I will try to reproduce the stages of dying described by the author in the sequence in which they occur (the author himself describes a theoretical model of dying, allowing a rearrangement of its events).

Inexpressibility

People who have experienced it characterize their experience as ineffable, i.e. inexpressible :
"It's a real challenge for me to explain all this to you because all the words I know are three-dimensional. At the same time, when I was going through this, I couldn't stop thinking: well, here we are, when I was going through geometry, I was always taught that there are only three dimensions, and I always believed that. But that's wrong. There are more."

Feelings of peace and tranquility

Many people describe extremely pleasant sensations and feelings during the first stages of their experience. *"At the moment of injury I felt a sudden pain, but then all the pain disappeared. I felt as if I were floating in a dark space. I felt nothing but peace, relief-exactly peace. I found that all my anxieties were gone and I thought how peaceful, good and there was no pain."*

Noise

Many reports mention all sorts of unusual auditory sensations at or before the time of death. Sometimes they are extremely unpleasant. Here are descriptions from different people: *"a very unpleasant buzzing sound coming from inside my head"; "a loud ringing, it could be described as a buzzing, and I was like in a spinning state"; "I started to hear some music, majestic music, really beautiful".*

A dark tunnel

Often at the same time as the noise effect there is a sensation of moving at very high speed through some dark space. Many different expressions are used to describe it: it has been described as a cave, a well, something through, a confined space, a tunnel, a chimney, a vacuum, a void, a drain, a valley, a cylinder.

"The first thing I heard-I want to describe it exactly as it happened-was a ringing, very rhythmic noise, something like: brrrrninnnnnnnng-brrrrninnng-brrrrnng, then I moved-you can think of it as something supernatural-through a long dark space. It was like a tunnel. I was moving and I kept hearing this ringing noise."

Outside the body

Before their near-death experiences, people did not differ in their attitude to this question from the average person. That is why the dying person is so amazed after he passes through a dark tunnel. Because he finds himself looking at his physical body as if he were an outside observer, a "third party". Emotional reactions to this state vary. Most people say that at first they experience a desperate desire to go back into their body, but don't know how to do it. Others report experiencing a very intense, panicky fear. Some describe a positive reaction to their condition. *" Look, I didn't even know I looked like this. You know, I'm used to only seeing myself in pictures or in the mirror, and in both cases it looks flat. But suddenly it turned out that I, or my body, was completely different-and I could see it. It took me a few minutes to recognize myself."*

In one or two cases that Dr. Moody met, dying people whose soul, mind, consciousness (or you can call it something else) had separated from the body said that after they came out they did not feel they had a bodily shell. They perceived themselves as "pure" consciousness. The author has chosen the term "spiritual body" to describe this phenomenon.

These properties of the spiritual body, which seem to be limitations, can also be seen as the absence of limitations. A person possessing a spiritual body is in a privileged position in relation to others: he can see them, hear them, but they do not see or hear him. Traveling in this state is made extremely easy. Physical objects do not constitute any obstacle, and travel from one place to another can be very rapid, almost instantaneous. In addition, the spiritual body, although it is not noticeable to those with physical bodies, is "something". Everyone agrees that it has a shape or outline (sometimes rounded or in the form of a shapeless cloud, and sometimes resembling the outline of a physical body) and even separate parts (protrusions or surfaces similar to arms, legs, head, etc.). Among the words and expressions used by different people were such as: fog, cloud, smoke-like, vapor, something transparent, colored cloud, something thin, a blob of energy, etc., and others. And finally, almost everyone notes that when one is outside the body, time does not exist.

"I remember being brought into the operating room. During that time, I left my body several times and came back into it. I could see my physical body directly from above. At the same time I was nevertheless in a body, but not in a physical body, but in another body, which I can characterize as a kind of energy. If I had to describe it in words, I would say that it was transparent and spiritual, as opposed to material objects. At the same time, it definitely had separate parts.

"The most striking part of the experience was that when my 'essence' stopped above my head, it was as if it was deciding whether to leave my body or return to it. It seemed that even then, time had not yet moved.

The nature of perception is similar and dissimilar to the perception of the physical body. As we have seen, kinesthesia, i.e. the internal state of the body, is absent as such. On the other hand, the sensations corresponding to physical hearing and vision remain unchanged in comparison with the physical state. " *When I wanted to discern someone at a distance, it seemed to me that a part of me, a kind of pull, was reaching out to what I wanted to see. At that time it seemed to me that whatever was happening anywhere on earth, I could be there if I wanted to be."*

"Hearing" inherent in the spiritual body can only be so named by analogy to that which takes place in the physical world, since most of the interviewees testify that they did not actually hear a physical sound or voice. Rather, they seemed to perceive the thoughts of those around them, and as we will see later, this same mechanism of direct transmission of opinions plays an important role in the later stages of the experience of death. *"I could see the people around me and understand everything they were saying. I couldn't hear them like I can hear you. It was like if I recognized what they were thinking, but it was only perceived through my mind, not through what they were saying. I already understood them a second before they opened their mouths to say anything."*

Meeting others

In many cases, the souls of people meet other "spiritual beings": their deceased relatives, friends, the sick who died shortly before. These beings were present with them to help and ease the dying into a new state or to inform them that the time of their death had not arrived and they should return to their physical body. In other similar cases, patients reported that they heard a voice telling them that they were not dead yet and would have to return again. Finally, these "spirit beings" may have an indeterminate form.

"When I was dead and in that void, I talked to people. But I couldn't say they were people. Every now and then I would talk to one of them, but I couldn't see anyone. When I tried to find out what was going on, I would always get a mental response from one of them that everything was fine. They never left my mind alone in the void.

"I heard a voice, but it was a non-human voice, and its perception was beyond the boundary of physical sensation. This voice was telling me that I had to go back, and I felt no fear of returning to my physical body".

A glowing creature

The most profound impression on people was the encounter with the luminous being. Identification varies from person to person and depends on the religious environment in which the person was formed, upbringing and personal faith. Christians believe that this light is Christ. People who do not believe simply say they saw a "luminous being". The love and warmth emanating from him cannot be described in words. The dying person feels complete relief and warmth, an irresistible attraction to this light.

Shortly after its appearance, this creature makes contact with the person who has come, as it can "pick up thoughts". The exchange of thoughts is almost instantaneous. The first thought it transmits is in the form of a question: Are you prepared for death? Are you ready to die? What have you done in your life that you can show me? At the same time, there is no accusation or threat in this question, everyone felt only an all-encompassing love and support coming from the light. Rather, it seems that this question is asked in order to bring the person to the path of knowledge about himself, to invite him to be frank.

"At first, when the light appeared, I didn't quite understand what was happening. It was beautiful, so brilliant, so radiant, but it didn't blind me at all. It was an unearthly light. It was the light of absolute understanding and perfect love." Mentally I heard: "Do you love me?" It wasn't said in the form of a definite question, but the meaning could be expressed as, "If you really love me, go back and finish in your life what you started." You see, this was a kind of test for me, the most significant one of my entire life. I felt really good-safe and surrounded by love. The love coming from him is something unimaginable, indescribable.

Pictures of the past

The initial appearance of the luminous being, the test and the questions without words are the prelude to the most striking and intense moment, during which it shows the person pictures, as if an overview of his life. It is obvious that the "luminous being" knows the whole life of the person and does not need any information. Its only intention is to provoke a reaction. While viewing such pictures from a person's life, the "luminous being" kept emphasizing the importance of love. *"The moments in which this was most strongly manifested were in connection with my sister. I have always been close to her, and he showed me several instances in which I was selfish toward my sister, and then several instances where I really showed her love and compassion. He pointed out to me that I should strive to help people, strive to be a better person."*

He also seemed to be interested in questions about knowledge. Each time he noted events related to the teachings and told me that I should continue to learn and that when he came for me again (by this time he had already told me that I would be coming back), the pursuit of knowledge would remain. He said it was an ongoing process, and I had a feeling it would continue even after death. *I* think he was trying to teach me as we went over the scenes of my life."

Boundary or limit

In some examples, patients reported that during their near-death experience they approached something that could be called a boundary or a limit: a body of water, a boat connecting two shores, a gray fog, a door, a fence stretching along a field, or simply a line. *"A bright light appeared before me. A mental or verbal question reached my consciousness: Do you want to die? I answered: I don't know. Then the white light said to me: Cross this line and you will know. I felt that there was a line ahead of me, though I did not see it. As soon as I crossed this line, I had an even more amazing feeling of peace, tranquility, no preoccupation.*

Return

In all interviewees, the first moments of their death are dominated by a frantic desire to return back to the body. But when the deceased reaches a certain stage of dying, they do not want to go back, especially if they have met a "luminous being". Others have felt that they "received permission" to live from God or a "luminous being," or because they were compelled to fulfill a mission. And in a few cases, people feel that the prayers or love of others, their loved ones, can bring them back, regardless of their own desire.

"I was by my aunt's side during her serious illness. Throughout her illness, someone in the family prayed for her recovery. Several times she stopped breathing, but we would bring her back. One time she looked at me and said: Joan, I have to go there, it's so beautiful. I want to stay there, but I can't while you pray for me to be with you. Please don't pray anymore. We stopped, and soon she died."

Impact on life

The experience had a very subtle, calming effect on the lives of these people. Many said that their lives had become deeper and more meaningful because their experience had made them more interested in ultimate philosophical questions. For example, one of these patients said that the state of her mind had become the primary concern, and that the care of the body came second - it was simply necessary to maintain a reasonable life. Another person feels it is now his duty on earth to learn the kind of love he felt in the matter of the "luminous being": can he love others in the same way? Many emphasize the importance of acquiring knowledge. "No matter what age you are, don't stop learning. I think learning is a process that goes on forever."

A new attitude toward death

Every single one of these survivors has expressed the same idea that they are no longer afraid of death. Death ceases to be frightening because the survivor no longer doubts that life does not cease with the death of the body. They offer analogies of death as an exit of consciousness to a higher level of being. A woman who met her relatives during her "dying" now compares death to "coming home." Others compared death to a pleasant event: waking up, being released from prison. *"Life is like a prison sentence. But in this state, we just don't realize what a prison our body is to us. Death is like a release, a release from prison. That's the best thing I could compare it to."*

Naturally, none of the people mentioned the common mythological picture of postmortem existence: heaven with pearly gates paved with gold, winged angels playing harps; no one spoke of hellfire and devils with pitchforks.

CHAPTER 4
LEGALIZING EUTHANASIA OR ASSISTED SUICIDE: THE ILLUSION OF SAFETY AND CONTROL

In 30 years, the Netherlands has moved from euthanasia of people who are terminally ill, to euthanasia of those who are chronically ill; from euthanasia for physical illness, to euthanasia for mental illness; from euthanasia for mental illness, to euthanasia for psychological distress or mental suffering-and now to euthanasia simply if a person is over the age of 70 and "tired of living". Dutch euthanasia protocols have also moved from conscious patients providing explicit consent, to unconscious patients unable to provide consent. Denying euthanasia or PAS in the Netherlands is now considered a form of discrimination against people with chronic illness, whether the illness be physical or psychological, because those people will be forced to "suffer" longer than those who are terminally ill. Non-voluntary euthanasia is now being justified by appealing to the social duty of citizens and the ethical pillar of beneficence. In the Netherlands, euthanasia has moved from being a measure of last resort to being one of early intervention. Belgium has followed suit and troubling evidence is emerging from Oregon specifically with respect to the protection of people with depression and the objectivity of the process.

Keywords: *acts, rejection of actions, death, intentions, termination of life, euthanasia, assisted suicide.*

Euthanasia is generally defined as an act undertaken only under the supervision of a physician that intentionally ends a person's life at his or her request [11, 12]. Therefore, the physician prescribes a lethal substance. "Physician-assisted suicide" (hereinafter referred to as suicide) on the one hand appears as a patient's decision to self-administer a lethal dose of a medication prescribed by a physician.

To date, the Netherlands, Belgium and Luxembourg have legalized euthanasia [13, 14]. Laws in the Netherlands and Luxembourg also allow euthanasia. In the United States, the states of Oregon and Washington legalized "physician-assisted suicide" in 1997 and 1999, respectively, but euthanasia remains illegal [15]. The situation in Montana currently remains unclear; a bill legalizing suicide was passed by the state legislature in 2010, but was recently overturned by the Senate State Law Committee.

In Holland, euthanasia and suicide were formally legalized in 2001 after a 30-year period of public debate [16]. Since the 1980s, guidelines and procedures for the control of euthanasia have been developed and adapted several times by the Royal Dutch Medical Association in collaboration with the national judiciary. Despite opposition from the Belgian Medical Association, Belgium legalized euthanasia in 2002, after 3 years of public debate that included members of government commissions. Luxembourg legalized euthanasia and suicide in 2009. In Switzerland, although not formally legalized, a law amendment was passed in the early 1900s that excludes suicide.

Euthanasia, however, is an illegal act [17]. A person commits suicide, may do so with the assistance of an assisted person as long as the assisted person has no self-interested motives and gains nothing personally from the death. Unlike other jurisdictions that require only physicians to perform euthanasia or assisted suicide, Switzerland allows more than just physicians to assist suicide.

In all of these jurisdictions, there are no safeguards, criteria or procedure for the implementation of controls in practice to ensure public order, and to prevent either the abuse or misuse of euthanasia [18]. Some criteria and procedures for euthanasia are common to all jurisdictions; others vary from country to country [19, 20]. In order to prevent the abuse of euthanasia, special care should be taken when legalizing euthanasia in countries that intend to legalize it. This review article examines the effectiveness of safeguards and "side effects" in the practice of euthanasia.

4.1. *Safeguards, their effectiveness*

In all legislative documents, a request for euthanasia or suicide must be voluntary, considered, informed, and enduring over time. The requestor must provide written consent and must be competent at the time the request is made. Despite these safeguards, more than 500 people in the Netherlands are put to sleep involuntarily every year. In 2005, a total of 2,410 deaths by euthanasia or suicide represents 1.7% of all deaths in the Netherlands. More than 560 people (0.4% of all deaths) were administered lethal substances without their explicit consent [27]. Out of every 5 patients, 1 is put to sleep without their explicit consent. Attempts to bring these cases to court have failed, suggesting that the judicial system has become more tolerant of such criminal acts over time [28].

In Belgium, the rate of involuntary rather than voluntary euthanasia of deaths (i.e. without explicit consent) is 3 times higher than in the Netherlands [38, 39]. "Involuntary euthanasia" includes situations in which the person has capacity but has not provided consent to "involuntary euthanasia, and situations in which the person is unable to give consent for reasons such as dementia or coma. A recent study showed that in the Flemish part of Belgium, 66 out of 208 cases of "euthanasia" (32%) occurred in the absence of a request or consent for euthanasia [17]. The reasons for terminating a person' life without obtaining consent were the following: patients being in coma (70% of cases) or dementia (21% of cases). In 17% of cases, physicians performed euthanasia without patient consent because they believed that euthanasia was "clearly in the patient's best interest" and, in 8% of cases, physicians believed that discussing euthanasia with the patient would be to the patient's detriment. These findings are consistent with a previous study in which 25 of 1644 sudden deaths were the result of euthanasia without explicit patient consent [38].

Figure 1. Schematic diagram of the structure of HIV infection.

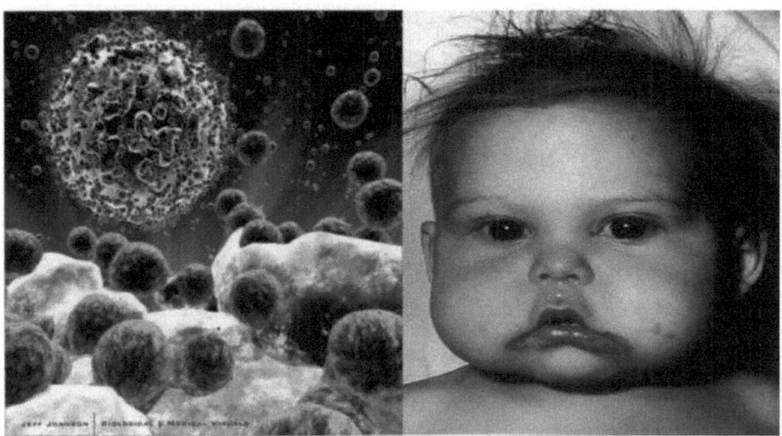

Figure 2. The photograph shows an infant with symptoms of Kwashiorkor disease - energy-protein malnutrition and vitamin B deficiency. Kwashiorkor disease is associated with inadequate protein intake, thinning hair, swelling, poor growth, and weight loss. Angular stomatitis is indicative of concomitant vitamin B deficiency.

Bypassing laws provides some evidence from social research on the "side effects" of euthanasia described by Keown [25,47]. So far, no cases of euthanasia have been found to be referred to the judiciary for further investigation in Belgium. In the Netherlands, 16 cases (0.21% of all recorded cases) were referred to the judiciary in the first 4 years after the euthanasia law came into force, with no euthanasia cases prosecuted [55]. In one case, a counselor who advises a terminally ill patient on how to commit suicide was acquitted [38]. Consequently, the enactment of the euthanasia law indicates a change in societal values following the legalization of euthanasia and assisted suicide. In 1987, the Royal Dutch Medical Association wrote in the preamble of its guidelines on euthanasia, "if there is no request from the patient, then the decision to end his life [legally] qualifies as murder or suicide, not euthanasia." In 2001, the association supported a new law that wrote the wish for an advance directive for euthanasia as acceptable, with representatives of the judicial system tolerating involuntary euthanasia [17,39,40]. However, decisions based on a request for advance disposition or a will may be ethically problematic because a request that does not coincide with the act cannot be evidence of the patient's will at the time of euthanasia.

In Oregon, although unbearable suffering that cannot be relieved by medication must be present in a terminal illness with a prognosis of less than 6 months to live, it is not a basic requirement for euthanasia to be performed (again recognizing that the concept of "unbearable suffering" is itself ambiguous). This definition allows physicians to provide assisted suicide without reference to the medical, psychological, social circumstances and concerns that typically underlie a request for assisted suicide. Physicians are required to indicate that palliative care is a viable alternative, but are not required to be knowledgeable about how to alleviate physical or emotional suffering. Until 2001, only adults in the Netherlands were allowed access to euthanasia or suicide. However, in 2001, the law allowed euthanasia for children aged 12 - 16 years, with parental permission for child death, although this age group generally constitutes a group of patients deemed unfit to make such a decision[5]. The law even allows doctors to proceed with euthanasia if there is disagreement between parents. By 2005, Groningen had adopted a protocol that authorizes euthanasia of newborns and young children who should have "no hope of a good quality of life" [30, 31]. In 2006, legislators in Belgium announced their intention to change the law to include euthanasia of infants, adolescents, and people with dementia or Alzheimer's disease [32].

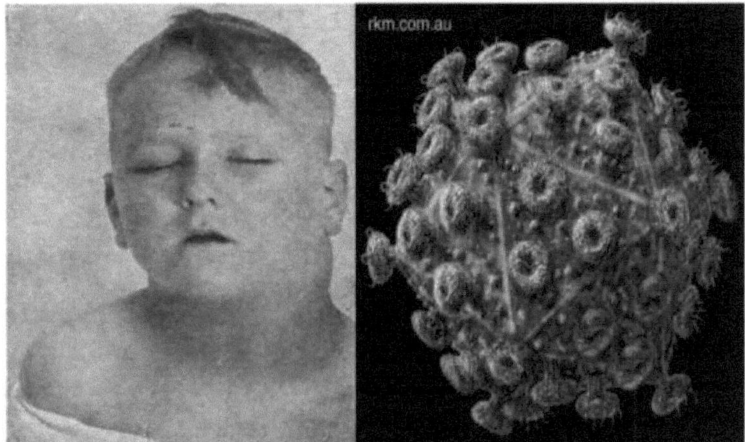

Figure 3. Photograph taken from the textbook Hodgkin's Disease in 1938.
Figure 4. Ag HIV (HIV infection antigen).   Statistics
shows that HIV-infected children have 1200 times higher risk of such diseases as: non-Hodgkin's lymphoma - , leiomyoma and leiomyosarcoma - 15%, leukemia - 6%, Kaposi's sarcoma - 5%, Hodgkin's lymphoma - 3%, carcinoma - 2%. Without treatment of HIV-infection, mortality increases by 40 - 70 %. Pneumocystis pneumonia occurs episodically in 80% of HIV-infected children.

In Belgium, specialists chose to ignore the requirement that, in the case of abandonment of terminally ill patients, an interval of 1 month must be observed from the time of the first request until euthanasia is performed. One specialist reported that his unit took into account the average time from patient admission to the time euthanasia was performed, seemingly in a "hopeless" situation patients had about 3.5 days [33]. This specialist argued that the underlying principle was beneficence. Initially, euthanasia in the Netherlands was, as a last resort, in the absence of other treatment options. Surprisingly, however, palliative care by a counselor is not mandatory in jurisdictions allowing euthanasia or assisted suicide, although uncontrolled pain and symptoms remain among the reasons for requesting euthanasia or suicide [34].

From 2002 to 2007 in Belgium, palliative care was performed by physician consultation (second opinion) in only 12 % of all euthanasia cases [39]. Palliative care by the medical team was performed in more than 65% of euthanasia admissions. In addition, palliative care services have been declining. In 2002, palliative care by the medical team was consulted in 19% of euthanasia cases, but by 2007 it had decreased to 9% of cases. Finding that in Belgium, legalization has been accompanied by significant improvements in palliative care in the country [25]. Other studies report a decline in palliative care [28,41]. It should be noted that legalization of euthanasia or suicide is not required in other countries, such as the United Kingdom, Australia, Ireland, France, and Spain, in which palliative care is more developed than in Belgium and the Netherlands.

There are other examples that the "social slippery slope" as a phenomenon does exist. In Switzerland, in 2006, the University Hospital in Geneva reduced its palliative care staff (1.5 to 2 full-time doctors) after the hospital decided to allow suicide, and the palliative care center was also closed. 15% of physicians in the Netherlands expressed concern that economic pressures might lead them to consider euthanasia for some of their patients; an already dying patient is put to sleep to free up a hospital bed [46]. There is evidence that involving physicians in palliative care would be made more difficult because providing palliative care requires competence and emotional and time commitment on the part of the clinician [47,48]. In the UK, at a parliamentary hearing on euthanasia a few years ago, a Dutch doctor argued that "we don't need palliative care, we practice euthanasia" [49]. Proponents of euthanasia generally ignore these concerns about the "social slippery slope" and have chosen to refute this "slippery slope" as an argument on the grounds that legalization of euthanasia and suicide has not resulted in an exponential increase in euthanasia or a disproportionate number of vulnerable individuals [56,57,58]. However, there is evidence that these claims are unreliable. The number of deaths by euthanasia in Flanders has doubled since 1998 [38]. Of the total number of deaths in this Flemish part of Belgium (population 6 million), 1.1%, 0.3%, and 1.9% occurred by euthanasia in 1998, 2001, and 2007, respectively [18] (about 620, 500, and 1040 people, respectively, in those years). Chambaere et al. [40] reported in their Canadian Medical Association report that in Belgium, euthanasia without patient consent decreased from 3.2% in 1998 to 1.8% in 2007. However, a closer review of the original study shows that the euthanasia rate decreased to 1.5% in 2001 and then increased again to 1.8% in 2007 [37].

In Holland, the overall euthanasia rate was 1.7% of all deaths in 2005, compared with 2.4% and 2.6% in 2001 and 1995, respectively, but not different since 1990, when the rate was 1.7% [57]. However, the Dutch government, citing official statistics, indicates a 13% increase in euthanasia in 2009 compared to 2008; euthanasia now accounts for 2% of all deaths. Given the growing numbers, the interest of institutions providing euthanasia (similar cases have been reported in Swiss assisted suicide thanks to the professionals of the Dignitas group). In

Oregon, although in some cases, the percentage of euthanasia is very low in relation to the population: 24 prescriptions were written in 1998 (16 of which resulted in death by -assisted suicide), 67 such cases were recorded in 2003 (43 of which resulted in death by suicide), and 89 similar cases were found in 2007 [50].

In Belgium, involuntary euthanasia services have decreased; they accounted for 3.2%, 1.5%, and 1.8% of all deaths in 1998, 2001, and 2007, respectively (1800, 840, and 990, respectively, patients in those years) [68]. In the Netherlands, the practice of euthanasia decreased from 0.7% in 2001 to 0.4% in 2005 [57]. The actual rate is probably higher due to the large number of unreported cases.

Baitin et al. [61] examined data from Oregon and the Netherlands and concluded , in contrast to other authors [68], that there is no evidence that vulnerable people, other than those with AIDS, are disproportionately sedated. "Vulnerable" was defined in this study as people such as the elderly, women, uninsured, people with low educational status, poor, disabled, or chronically ill, younger than the age of most survivors with mental disorders including depression, racial or ethnic minority.

George and Finley challenged in their study that vulnerability to associated suicide or euthanasia cannot be attributed to race, gender, or socioeconomic status. Other characteristics such as emotional state, response to loss, personality type, and sense of burden are also important [62]. For example, one study found that the more physicians knew about palliative care, the less they practiced euthanasia and assisted suicide [63].

Two recent studies contradict the findings of colleagues. Chambérété et al. state that voluntary and involuntary euthanasia occurs predominantly among patients 80 years and older who were comatose or demented [50]. According to them, these patients "do not fit the description of vulnerable patient populations at risk of end of life without request." The researchers concluded that "peer attention should be paid to protecting these patient groups from such practices." In another study, two factors were significantly associated with nurses managing patients' lives by dispensing narcotic drugs in the absence of an explicit request from patients aged 80 years and older [62].

4.2. Understanding the reasons for euthanasia

What can be done when palliative care does not alleviate suffering? A palliative care specialist who has worked in the Netherlands with people who have requested euthanasia and associated suicide provides a taxonomy for understanding the reasons behind requests for euthanasia.

Requests can be classified into five categories [64]:

* Fear about what will happen in the future
* Experiencing burnout from a relentless disease
* Having the desire and need to manage the disease
* Experiencing depression
* Experiencing extreme suffering, including dull aches and other symptoms

These strategies are available for decision making for severe refractory symptoms, for treating depression, and for dealing with the fear that some people associate with a tomorrow with a terminal illness. Approximately 10 - 15% of pain and other physical symptoms (e.g., shortness of breath and delirium) cannot be controlled on the first and second attempt. For these symptoms, there is the option of palliative sedation. Palliative sedation is defined as "the controlled use of medication designed to induce a state of diminished or lack of awareness (unawareness) of the fact that the burden of otherwise intractable suffering is being alleviated in a manner that is ethically acceptable to the patient, family and health care providers and to patients who are about to die" [65]. Its meaning is not to hasten death, which distinguishes it from euthanasia. The goal is to achieve comfort with the lowest dose of sedation possible to start (usually with a midazolam infusion rather than an opioid) and then move to the lightest level of sedation possible. Some patients are thus willing to achieve comfort with light levels of sedation, allowing them to continue interacting with family; in others, comfort is achieved only with deep levels of sedation.

Studies have shown that dignity and hope are lost and, taking on a sense of burden, patients proceed to seek euthanasia and assisted suicide [67-70, 74]. Strategies to enhance dignity, drawing on empirical studies that have explored the concept of dignity in palliative care, have been shown in [75].

Given the effectiveness of palliative care, including palliative sedation for patients with persistent symptoms, the only remaining issue is the legalization of "on demand" euthanasia and assisted suicide when there is no end of illness or when a person is tired of life or has a mental illness. Legalizing euthanasia and assisted suicide in these circumstances is most relative and would have serious consequences over time, including changes in societal values and suicide prevention decisions, because people who wish to take their own lives would then have that right.

CHAPTER 5
EPIDEMIOLOGIC AND CLINICAL FEATURES
COURSE OF HIV INFECTION ASSOCIATED WITH MYCOBACTERIUM LEPRAE IN PATIENTS WITH
MYCOBACTERIUM LEPRAE-ASSOCIATED HIV INFECTION IN PATIENTS (MEDICAL, SOCIAL AND CLINICAL ASPECTS)

The findings from article review are representative of all cases of HIV/M. leprae co-infection living in Rio de Janeiro as the study was based on a non probability haphazard sample from a single center for leprosy treatment in the city of Rio de Janeiro. As a referral center, the clinic receives more frequently patients with severe presentations of the disease such as type 1 reactions. Still, the amount of missing data, especially related with the characteristics of the HIV infection, made further analysis difficult. However, the 92 co-infectedpatients in the present article review make up the largest HIV/M. leprae cohort under analysis in the international literature. The authors strongly believe that the majority of the patients co-infected with HIV/M. leprae are in the state of Rio de Janeiro. The present article review shows that an increasing number of co-infected patients have been admitted over the last 15 years at the leprosy outpatients clinic. In contrast, the burden of leprosy and AIDS has declined in Rio de Janeiro over the same period of time. Co-infectedpatient admissions have steadily increased over the last years at this referral center. Most patients were men, with a mean age of 32.3 years and presenting with the paucibacillary form of leprosy. The use of antiretroviral therapy (ART) was the only factor associated with type 1 reaction. Most patients were living in the metropolitan area and the north sub area of Rio de Janeiro City.

Keywords: *immuno deficiency syndrome, erythema nodosum leprosum, type 1 lepra reaction.*

A number of studies have demonstrated a causal relationship between socioeconomic factors and the spread of infectious diseases. Such a detailed study of factors can explain the geographical and socio-demographic patterns of leprosy spread and the possible clustering of different infectious diseases within the same geographical area or among the affected population. Thus, the study of lepra involves the study of various factors such as various tropical diseases, HIV/AIDS in the context of poverty and marked socioeconomic and geographic heterogeneity. Since the beginning of the AIDS epidemic in the early eighties, the role of co-infection in combination with tropical diseases, tuberculosis, leishmaniasis and malaria have been studied in Brazil [90, 91].

As recently shown by a study in the Lancet, with appropriate infectious disease control as a key factor in preventing epidemics on a global scale, it is possible to manage various coinfections, and it is necessary to provide optimal care for those already infected with HIV/AIDS [92]. Despite evidence that HIV infection can alter the natural course of lepra [93], there are few epidemiologic data on HIV/Mycobacterium leprae coinfection published in the literature [94].

Leprosy occurs mainly in countries in tropical and subtropical regions of the world. According to reports from the WHO, 105 countries reported 219,075 new cases of co-infection during 2011 [95], although there has been a downward trend in overall prevalence and first-time cases in recent years, leprosy remains a pressing public health problem in Brazil. In 2011, the prevalence rate was 1.54 cases per 10,000 inhabitants and 33,955 new cases of leprosy were detected throughout the country [96].

In addition, HIV infection remains one of the most serious public health problems due to its pandemic nature and high morbidity and mortality in areas where effective therapies remain elusive. With an estimated 2.5 million people infected with HIV in 2011 and 34 million people detected with symptoms of HIV infection at the end of 2011 in Brazil, the AIDS epidemic has stabilized over the past 10 years. In 2011, the incidence rate was 20.2 cases per 100,000 inhabitants, with 38,776 new AIDS cases registered throughout the country [97].

To date, there is no reliable estimate of the number of AIDS/Lepro co-infected patients according to official publications. However, analysis of documentary and archival data confirms outbreaks of both diseases in the poorest regions of Brazil, as well as in sub-Saharan African and Southeast Asian foci of this co-infection. In the last decade, the attention of the scientific community has been drawn to outbreaks of leprosy and HIV co-infection type 1 leprosy reaction after the initiation of combination antiretroviral therapy [94] of leprosy co-infected patients. Those affected by HIV are at higher risk of developing type 1 leprosy reactions, and it is also well known that leprosy reactions result from an immunologic shift in the patient at the level of inflammation and/or cell-mediated immunity, which in turn can lead to accelerated nerve damage and severe physical disabilities.

To evaluate the clinical and epidemiological patterns of HIV infection/mycobacterium leprae in co-infected patients in Brazil, data on patients with leprosy were obtained by excerpting from a reference and information center located in the city of Rio de Janeiro, summarized and analyzed. Outpatient charts with addresses of local residents were used to evaluate the geographical distribution of co-infected patients. In addition, comorbidities associated with type 1 leprosy reactions were evaluated, as well as sociodemographic and clinical data from medical records.

The city of Rio de Janeiro is the main and most important municipality in Brazil, with a population of about 6,320,446.

Although the second wealthiest city in the country (the first was São Paulo), Rio de Janeiro has suffered from entrenched socioeconomic inequalities [96], a large proportion of its population still lives in difficult living conditions [97]. The city of 160 neighborhoods has historically been divided into four regions: south, north, west, and central. According to the last census of 2010, in Brazil, Rio de Janeiro had a population of 15,989,929 people, the vast majority of whom (96.7%) lived in urban areas, especially in the larger neighborhoods of the capital city of Rio de Janeiro. Rio de Janeiro is divided into 5 meso-regions, namely South, North, Northwest and Central. The Leprosy Reference and Information Center is a center of excellence for leprosy diagnosis, treatment and care, and contact tracing. Under the auspices of the Brazilian Ministry of Health, the evaluation of HIV/lepro co-infected patients began in 1989.

5.1.   *Patient characteristics at the time of diagnosis*

From January 1989 to December 2011, 92 leprosy patients with HIV positive serology were referred to the leprosy clinic center. Most of these patients (83/92; 90%) had a diagnosis of HIV established prior to the diagnosis of leprosy and 9 (10%) patients were diagnosed with HIV at the time of leprosy detection. Out of 92 patients, fifty two (57%) were male, the mean age at the time of diagnosis was 32.3 years, the age of all patients ranged from (18-72) years. Marital status and education were available for 86 of the 92 patients included in the database. The vast majority (70/86; 81%) were unmarried (single and divorced). The majority (66/86; 77%) had 1 to 8 years of formal schooling, while 21% (18/86) had attended school for more than 8 years and 2% (2/86) had never attended school.

Although the vast majority of patients were classified as paucibacillary carriers (71/92; 77%) because they had a bacilloscopic index of zero, nearly half (41/92; 45%) of patients had a negative   leprosy test (<5 mm).

Of the 92 patients included in the study, 33 (36%) patients were hospitalized for leprosy and at the time of diagnosis, 32 (97%) patients had type 1 and one patient type 2 leprosy reactions. Ridley and Jopling proposed the criteria used to classify the 59 patients who were not leprosy positive as follows: two (3%) patients were classified as tuberculoid type of reaction; 33 (56%) patients were classified as borderline tuberculoid type; four (7%) patients were classified as borderline inflammatory; five (8%) patients were classified as borderline lepromatous reaction; two (3%) patients were classified as lepromatous type of reaction; 11(19%) patients were classified as indeterminate type, and two (3%) patients had neural signs of clinical leprosy.

5.2. Discussion

The results of the review article are by no means representative of all typical cases of HIV/Mycobacterium leprae co-infection among residents of Rio de Janeiro, as the study by the foreign authors was based on the probability of random sampling from a single leprosy treatment center in the city of Rio de Janeiro. As a reference center, the clinic treats predominantly patients with severe manifestations of the disease, such as type 1 leprosy reactions. Still, the amount of missing data related to the peculiarities of the course of HIV infection was obtained during further detailed analysis of patients registered in the database of this center.

Until 2013, the 92 co-infected patients in this review article constitute the largest cohort of HIV/Mycobacterium leprae patients according to the results of studies in the foreign literature. The foreign authors are convinced that the majority of co-infected patients are HIV/mycobacterium leprae in the state of Rio de Janeiro were taken from the center's database, and were identified through referrals to the leprosy center. This literature review shows that an increasing number of co-infected patients with leprosy have been detected during the last 15 years when presenting to the polyclinic. Over a similar period of observation, the number of leprosy and AIDS cases detected has decreased in Rio de Janeiro. One possible explanation for this is that the recent increase in leprosy outbreaks since 1997, and the ability to access antiviral therapy at the leprosy center have become available to all patients

AIDS in Brazil.

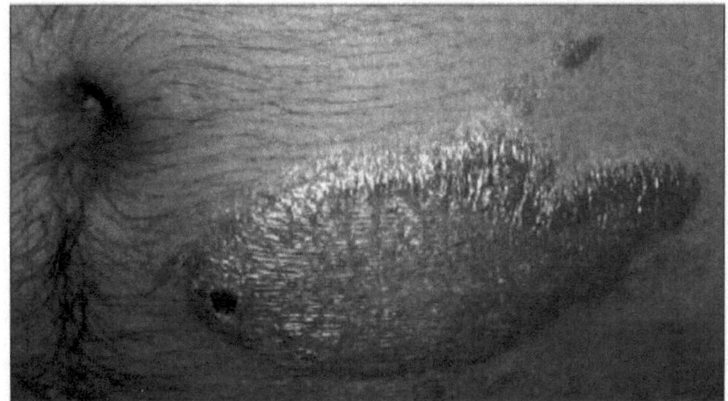

Figure 5. Erythematous plaques in a case of borderline tuberculoid leprosy type 1.

Some authors have suggested that the initiation of therapy is associated with the clinical picture of leprosy. Thus, the appearance of clinical signs of leprosy in persons with HIV infection is not considered a manifestation of immune suppression because they are markers of immune remodeling. Although HIV infection was expected to increase the incidence of multibacillary forms of lepra, this review suggests that HIV/Mycobacterium leprae in co-infected patients may be one manifestation of clinical forms of lepra. In fact, the results of patient referral showed a higher percentage of patients with the bacillary form of leprosy. Bacillus Paucibacillary leprosy is characterized by a strong cellular immune response with skin lesions contained as well-organized granulomas. It is hypothesized that the major antigenic stimuli associated with the gradual recovery of immune competence after initiation of lepra therapy may be associated with the appearance of granuloma and the subsequent appearance of tuberculoid skin reaction and nerve lesions.

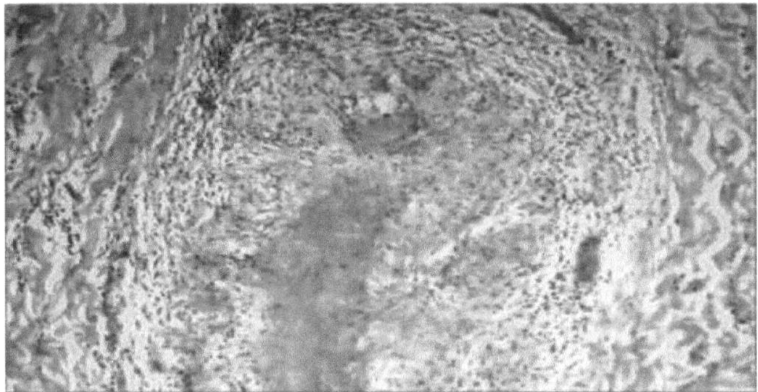

Figure 6. Caseous granulomas along the neurovascular bundle with a nerve infiltration in type 1 lepra (x400).

Lepra type 1 reactions are secondary to increased cellular immunity and delayed-type hypersensitivity to Mycobacterium leprae. Lepra-specific antiviral treatment is known to be associated with a dramatic viral load in HIV-infected individuals, whereas a decrease and subsequent increase in CD4 T cells, is a key marker of partial recovery of immune function. To fully clarify whether the high frequency of type 1 leprosy reaction is a response to diagnosis, as evidenced by the studies of most foreign authors, or is a consequence of immunologic recovery provoked by the use of treatment, further research in this scientific field is needed. Nevertheless, treatment initiation has been reported to be associated with activation of the subclinical course of lepra infection and exacerbation of pre-existing leprosy lesions. As an example, treatment utilization was the only independent factor associated with the presence of type 1 lepra reaction at the time of diagnosis. The socio-demographic characteristics of co-infected patients at their first visit to the specialized center presented here were similar to those observed among cases identified in Brazil nationwide. The national disease-related database shows a higher concentration of male patients between 30 and 59 years of age, as found in this observational study. Of the patients under 15 years of age were a minority of those hospitalized in the clinic, although this category represented 3.4% of all new leprosy cases in the state of Rio de Janeiro in 2010. This is explained by the low incidence of pediatric AIDS in Brazil (8.1/100,000 cases in 2010).

5.3. *Leprosy type 2 leprosy in an immunocompromised HIV-infected patient (based on literature review)*

Leprosy, also known as Hansen's disease, is a chronic disease caused by Mycobacterium leprae. Lepra bacteria tend to attack peripheral nerve endings, with the formation of characteristic deformities or type 1 or type 2 delayed leprosy reactions, which are major causes of morbidity. Type 2 leprosy reactions are immunologically mediated Gell or Coombs Type III hypersensitivity reactions. It is expressed in patients with lepromatous and borderline leprosy before, during, and less frequently after drug therapy for leprosy [98, 99]. Human immunodeficiency virus in HIV-infected patients also correlates with the presence of leprosy, as a rule, lepromatous type 1 reactions are present, which is confirmed by numerous publications of foreign authors. This review article presents one of the forms of leprosy - immune system weakening syndrome [100, 101], proving that leprosy reactions of type 2 very rarely occur in HIV-infected patients. To date, there is still no clear explanation of the reasons for this phenomenon [102]. In the last decade, despite numerous publications on the presence of type 1 leprosy reactions in HIV-infected patients with leprosy, cases of type 2 leprosy reactions have occurred less frequently in such patients. This review article presents a clinical case of acquired immunodeficiency syndrome (AIDS) with lepromatous leprosy, recurrent tuberculous lymphadenitis and lepromatous reaction type 2, manifested as leprosy nodular erythema, probably due to a positive precipitation reaction for filariasis [103], due to its relative rarity.

Clinical case

We present a clinical case: a 35-year-old man with recurrent episodes of high fever without diurnal temperature fluctuations, with red raised lesions over the skin for the past 1 year. The lesions were mainly on the face, ears, upper torso, and upper extremities. The patient had six such episodes of disease in the past year. He also complained of bilateral knee joint pain in 1 week without any swelling or limitation of motion.

The patient has received antiretroviral therapy for the past 1 year: zidovudine, lamivudine, and efavirenz. He had inguinal lymphadenitis 7 months ago, fine-needle aspiration cytology was performed, which showed tuberculous lymphadenitis, and antituberculosis treatment was prescribed. The patient is now taking isoniazid 300 mg, rifampicin 450 mg, and ethambutol 825 mg. Examination of the febrile patient revealed emaciation and weight loss of 18.5 kg/m^2. Bilateral thickening was found on the arms and legs on the right ulnar surface, and in the peroneal nerve area. Examination revealed erythematous nodules on the face, upper extremities, upper trunk, and ears (Figs. 7, 8). On palpation, nerve soreness, testicular edema, lymphadenopathy, and ocular pain or photophobia. Laboratory investigations showed severe anemia with hemoglobin (HB) 4.4 g/% and mean erythrocyte volume 3700 cells/mm^3, while leukocyte count was normal. The absolute number of SI4-lymphocytes is 90 cells/µL, enzyme-linked immunosorbent assay (ELISA) was performed for filariasis antigen, which was positive. Liver and renal tests, chest radiography, bilateral knee joint radiography, and general urinalysis were within normal limits. A pharyngeal swab for streptococcal culture showed no growth of organisms, Vidal tests for typhoid fever and microscopy for malaria parasites were negative.

Smear from the affected skin revealed 6+ acid-fast bacteria (Fig. 9). Biopsy from the nodule showed superficial and deep granulomatous inflammation with accumulation of neutrophils and nuclear debris around the affected vessels (Figure 10). Leprosy stains showed fragmentary analysis. Based on the above, the diagnosis of AIDS, lepromatous type 2 lepra with lepromatous reaction manifesting as in tuberculous lymphadenitis, filariasis was made.

The patient was treated with clofazimine (50 mg daily and monthly, controlled dose 300 mg, rifampicin 150 mg monthly, ofloxacin 200 mg twice daily, thalidomide 100 mg daily, and diethylcarbamazine 100 mg three times daily with iron preparations). The patient's condition improved dramatically and the lesions disappeared within 1 week. The patient was not found to have any lepromatous reaction during follow-up examinations.

Figure 7. Clinical picture showing erythematous-papulo-nodular lesions on the extensor surfaces of the forearm and hands.

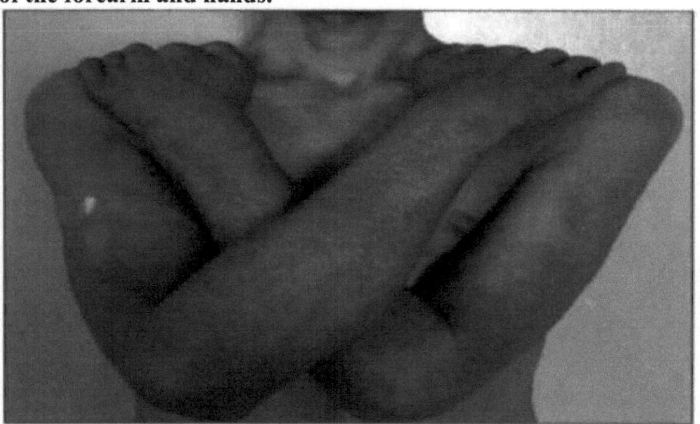

Figure 8. Erythematous plaques with indistinct edges on the *posterior* border of *the arms and shoulders.*

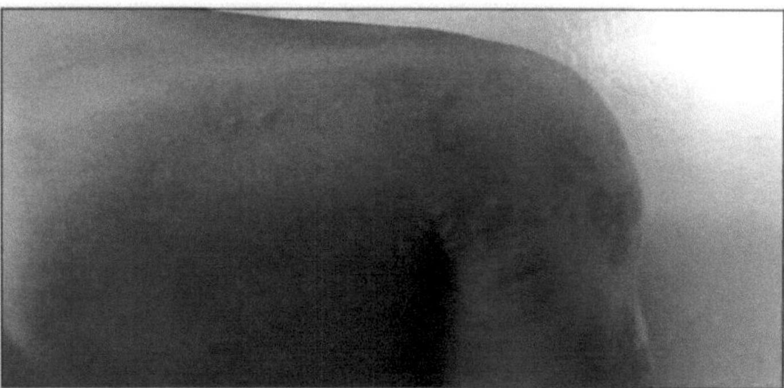

Figure 9. Examination of the skin smear showed 6+ acid-fast bacilli.

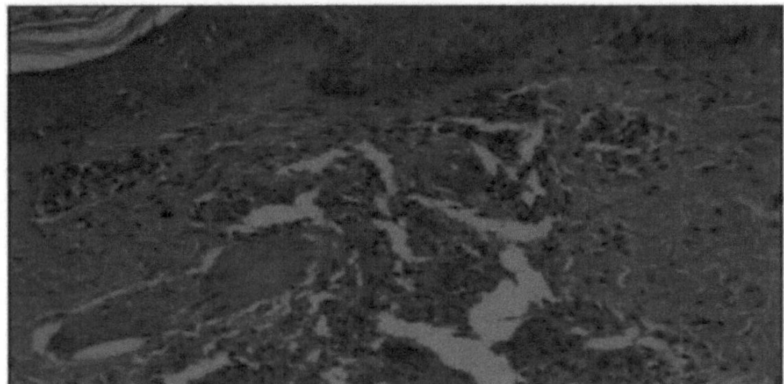

Figure 10. Histopathology shows superficial and deep granulomatous inflammation of neutrophils around vessels. Several foci with fragments of sputum microscopy (×100 magnification).

Leprosy is a chronic disease of infection of various body tissues with Mycobacterium leprae. Unfortunately, leprosy is endemic in India. India is also endemic to AIDS and hence there is a relatively high probability of the two of these diseases occurring together. In a study by Vinay et al, the prevalence of leprosy in patients was 5.22 per 1000 person-years (95% confidence interval 2.25- 10.28) [104] patients affected by AIDS and leprosy usually present Type 1 leprosy reactions, usually looks like a type of immune system recovery from the disease (AIDS) [105, 106]. Rarely, patients affected by lepromatous or borderline leprosy are found with Type 2 leprosy reactions. Type 2 leprosy reactions are a systemic inflammatory reaction in which immune complexes can form in any organ or tissue, and can be of a diverse nature [107]. Neuritis, orchitis, uveitis, periostitis, lymphadenitis, and glomerulonephritis may occur less frequently. Vinay et al, reported a case of eight patients in whom three had type 2 leprosy reactions. Similarly, Pai et al, reported cases of 11 patients coinfected with

HIV and leprosy in whom two patients had type 2 leprosy reactions. The literature review found two more case reports of patients with HIV and leprosy coinfection, which reported that type 2 leprosy reactions can be provoked by intercurrent infection, stress, pregnancy, lactation period, and various drugs. There have been published reports of filariasis provoking infection type 2 leprosy reactions in India. AIDS cases of tuberculous lymphadenitis with type 2 leprosy reactions manifesting as filariasis are occasionally encountered. Filariasis infection has been diagnosed with 98% sensitivity for both (Brugian and Bancroftian) types of filariasis [108]. The reason for the positive reaction for filariasis in this patient, could have been due to concealment of the case of his treatment for filariasis infection. India, being a country endemic for HIV infection, leprosy and infections such as tuberculosis and filariasis; the simultaneous presence of any of these can alter the course of treatment and blur the clinical course, creating diagnostic and therapeutic difficulties.

CHAPTER 6
HISTORICAL AND CLINICAL ASPECTS OF PORPHYRIA.
THE IMPORTANCE OF IRON IN THE DISRUPTION OF HEME BIOSYNTHESIS

Porphyrias are rare disorders that affect mainly the skin or nervous system and may cause abdominal pain. These disorders are usually inherited, meaning they are caused by abnormalities in genes passed from parents to children. When a person has a porphyria, cells fail to change body chemicals called porphyrins and porphyrin precursors into heme, the substance that gives blood its red color. The body makes heme mainly in the bone marrow and liver. Bone marrow is the soft, spongelike tissue inside the bones; it makes stem cells that develop into one of the three types of blood cells-red blood cells, white blood cells, and platelets.

1841 - The term 'porphyrin comes from the Greek word, porphyus, meaning reddish-purple. It was first thought that the reddish color of blood was from iron. One early scientist performed an experiment to prove that this was not the case. He washed dried blood with concentrated sulfuric acid to free the iron. He then treated it with alcohol and the resulting iron free residue took on a reddish purple color though it contained no iron compound.

Keywords: *porphyrias, hemoglobin, red blood cells, heme, protoporphyrin, red pigment.*

Relevance. Porphyria, a rare disorder affecting mainly the skin or nervous system, can cause abdominal pain. These disorders are usually inherited, meaning they are caused by abnormalities in genes, passed from parents to children. In the human body, heme is produced mainly in the bone marrow and in the liver. Bone marrow is a soft, sponge-like tissue within the bones; which causes stem cells to differentially develop into one of three types of blood cells-erythrocytes, white blood cells, and platelets [109].

The process of stem cell transformation is called heme biosynthesis. One of eight enzymes controls each step of the process. The human body has a problem, due to heme, if any of the enzymes are at low levels, called a deficiency. Porphyrins and heme precursors then build up in the body and cause disease. Heme is a red pigment made up of iron bound by a chemical called protoporphyrin. Heme has important functions in the body. The largest amount of heme is in the form of hemoglobin found in red blood cells and bone marrow [110].

The most common porphyrias are inherited disorders. Scientists have identified genes responsible for all eight enzymes of heme biosynthesis. The most common porphyrias are the result of inheriting an abnormal gene, also called a gene mutation from a single parent. Some porphyrias, such as congenital erythropoietic porphyria, hepatoerythropoietic porphyria, and erythropoietic protoporphyria, occur when a person inherits two abnormal genes, one from each parent. The likelihood of a person inheriting an abnormal gene or genes in the next generation, depends on the type of porphyria. Porphyria of the cutanea tarda type, is usually an acquired disorder triggered by external factors other than hereditary porphyria, which can lead to enzyme deficiency. This type of porphyria can be caused by:

•   with high levels of iron;

•   with alcohol or estrogen use;

•   smoking;

•   chronic hepatitis C-a long-term liver disease that causes inflammation, or liver tumors;

•   The HIV virus that causes AIDS;

•   abnormal genes associated with   hemochromatosis are the most a common form of iron overload disease that causes the human body to absorb too much iron [111]. For all other types of porphyria, the symptoms of the disease can be caused by:

•   by drinking alcohol;
•   smoking;
•   the use of certain medications or hormones;
•   by exposure to sunlight;
•   with stress;
•   dieting and starvation.

6.1. Erythropoietic protoporphyria.

People with erythropoietic protoporphyria are recommended beta-carotene or cysteine to increase tolerance to sunlight, although these drugs do not reduce porphyrin levels. Experts recommend avoidance of viral hepatitis A and B vaccinations and avoidance of alcohol to prevent liver failure in patients with porphyria. A health care provider may use liver transplantation or various combinations of medications to treat patients who develop liver failure. Unfortunately, liver transplantation cannot correct the primary defect, which is the persistent overproduction of protoporphyrin in the red bone marrow. Successful bone marrow transplant surgeries can cure erythropoietic protoporphyria. Medical professionals only consider bone marrow transplantation if the disease is severe and leads to secondary liver disease [112].

6.2.   *Congenital erythropoietic porphyria and hepatoerythropoietic porphyria*

People with congenital erythropoietic porphyria or hepatoerythropoietic porphyria may need surgery to remove the spleen or blood transfusions to treat anemia. The surgeon removes the spleen in the hospital and the patient receives general anesthesia. In a blood transfusion, the patient receives blood through an intravenous catheter (IV) inserted into a vein. A technician performs the procedures at the blood transfusion center, and the patient does not need anesthesia [113].

6.3. From the history of porphyria

In 1874, Dr. J. Schultz described the case of a 33-year-old male weaver who suffered from excessive skin sensitivity, enlarged spleen, and reddish colored urine since infancy. The physician called the condition he identified pempigus Ieprosus. This is most likely the first description of a case of protoporphyria. The disease was later named after Dr. Schultz.

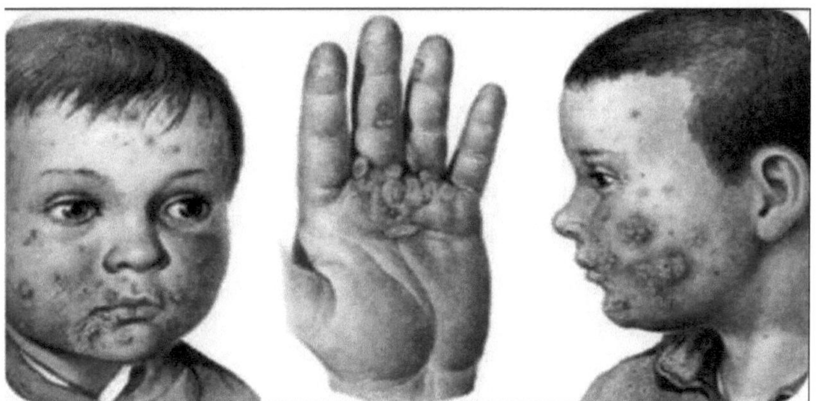

**Figure 11. A case of protoporphyria - first described in 1874
Dr. Schultz.**

In 1898 - McCall Anderson described two brothers with sunburned exposed skin. The disease was so severe that they lost part of their ears and nose. The patients were found to have red-colored urine [114].

In 1913, Dr. Friedrich Meyer Betz injected himself with hematoporphyrin to determine its photodynamic effects. The doctor soon discovered that his skin was sensitive to the action of sunlight, which was extremely painful, the photosensitivity lasting several months. In the photo of Dr. Betz, the photosensitivity lasted only a few hours after he injected himself with the drug, you can see his severely swollen face. He was unrecognizable until the tumor shrank (115).

In 1923 - A. E. Garrod first noted that hematoporphyria was, in fact, an inherited metabolic disease, as stated in his manuscript, an inborn error of metabolism. The term "inborn errors" of metabolism were first used for a group of inherited metabolic disorders by this scientist [116].

In 1937, Dr. Jan Waldenstrom suggested that the name of the disease was due to a disorder of porphyrin metabolism, so it should be considered porphyria rather than hematoporphyria. Using aldehyde, Paul Ehrlich's reagent, Dr. Waldenstrom identified 103 patients with acute porphyria by testing their urine, which was stained red. He found that asymptomatic family members of these patients also had a similar urine reaction that was detected when even small amounts of barbiturates and sulfonal were ingested.

In southeastern Turkey, between 1956 and 1961, an epidemic of *Porphyria cutanea tarda (PCT)* was reported. Apparently in 1954, the Turkish government distributed a shipment of wheat seeds that had been treated with fungicides containing 10% hexachlorobenzene (HCB). As many as 5,000 workers were reported to be affected by *porphyria cutanea tarda* because they were involved in the fungicide seed treatment. These workers showed symptoms of PCT as early as 1956. The government stopped the use of HCB-containing fungicide in 1959, so PCT outbreaks died out by 1961.

Researchers from the clinic analyzed the food history of the victims and found that 10% hexachlorobenzene was the cause of acquired PCT [117].

Acute intermittent porphyria is an autosomal dominant metabolic disorder that has various psychiatric manifestations. In acute intermittent porphyria, there is a breakdown in the biosynthetic pathway due to deficiency of uroporphobilinogen synthetase (porphobilinogen deaminase), resulting in overproduction of porphyrin precursors.

6.4. Clinical cases of porphyria

Six cases of porphyria described in 1990ˢ by the staff of Assam Medical College, Dibrugarh, all the patients were in the Department of Psychiatry on different occasions during one year: from January 1997 to December 1997. The report presents some of these clinical cases.

Case 1. Ms. M., a 35-year-old housewife and mother of two children, graduated from a rural middle class, working-class family. The woman was transferred on August 16, 1997, from Ward's medical ward with a diagnosis of hysteria due to her unconstructive behavior and slurred speech. She was admitted to the hospital room on August 12, 1997, in a semi-conscious state following repeated episodes of generalized tonic-clonic seizures, with no positive family history. Three months earlier, the patient had a similar seizure for which she had been taking phenytoin sodium, which provoked the above symptoms. Neurologic evaluation revealed peripheral neuropathy of all four limbs, XI and XII cranial nerves, paralysis, slurred speech. The patient was delirious. Her saturated urine color raised suspicion of porphyria. There was no abdominal pain. Urinary porphobilinogen showed a titer of 1:80.

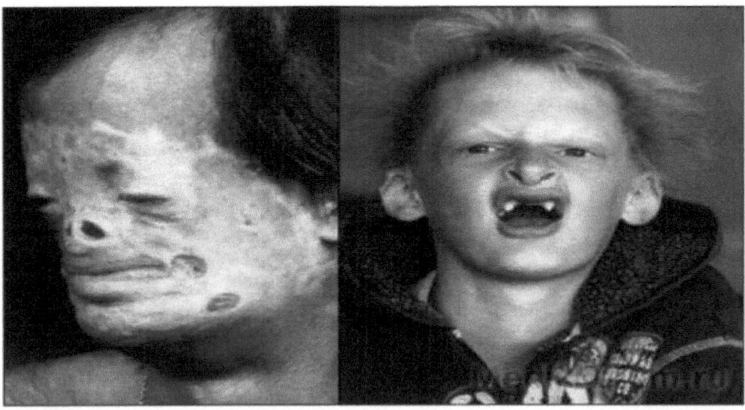

Figures 12, 13. **Clinical cases of porphyria.** *According to Dr. David Dolphin, a well-known porphyria specialist, the patient is adversely affected by even weak sunlight. Skin damage can be so severe that the nose or fingers can completely collapse. The lips and gums may shrink considerably while the teeth remain normal in size, resulting in an animal-like jaw with fangs. Porphyria patients may also experience increased hair growth.*

Case 2. Mrs. K, a 16-year-old girl, was referred by a physician on September 6, 1997, from a rural area with an aggravated family history and a history of psychiatric illness. She was admitted with complaints of insomnia, irritability, fits of aggression, and was treated with *chloroquin* for fever that had been present for 20 days. On examination, the girl had no symptoms of fever and complained of occasional abdominal pain. On physical examination, no abnormalities were found except for paroxysmal tachycardia. But on psychiatric evaluation, the patient presented with fear and panic attacks; a urine test for porphobilinogen showed a titer of 1:80, and Porphyria was suspected [118].

Case 3. Miss A., a 38-year-old housewife and mother of three children, from a middle-class urban family, was noted to have stable premorbid signs of porphyria with no concomitant family history but transient psychosis for 3 months. The patient was referred as in a case of "hysteria" to a psychiatrist with a history of dizziness and loss of consciousness. On admission, the patient had atonic seizures and autonomic lability in the form of paroxysmal tachycardia, sweating and anxiety with depression. Later, when she had severe pain and abdominal bloating with vomiting, porphyria was suspected, which was confirmed by a high titer of 1:10 porphobilinogen in a series of urine samples. On ultrasound, the findings signs of cholecystitis and cholelithiasis [119].

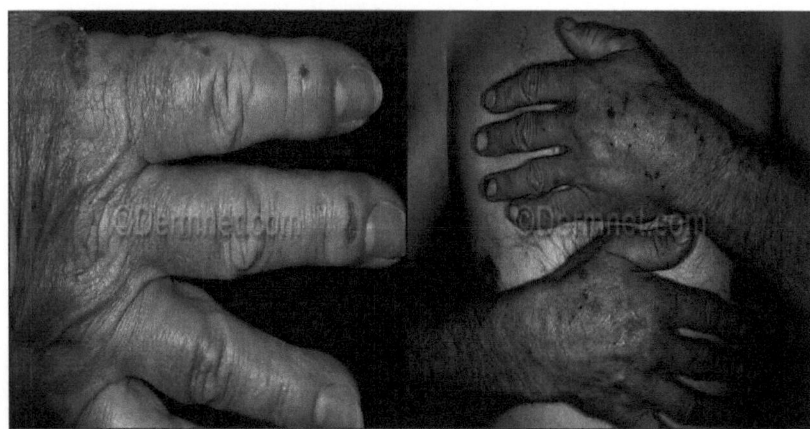

Figures 14, 15. Cases of erythropoietic protoporphyria. *Dolphin suggests that vampire bloodsuckers were also victims of porphyria and "sought to alleviate the symptoms of their terrible disease" in the Middle Ages by consuming large volumes of blood, which was the only way a person could obtain extra hemoglobin. Porphyria patients were desperate to get blood because the lack of hemoglobin caused death. Although the effect of hemoglobin entering the blood through the walls of the stomach is extremely small.*

Case 4. Mr. N., a 32-year-old married man, a rural cultivator with an aggravated family history, was admitted with a history of forgetfulness, weakness, poor digestion, insomnia, deterioration in social status, behavioral abnormalities, and generalized tonic-clonic seizures for a month and a half. He had never been treated for the seizures, although they had been present for 5 years. The patient was prescribed phenytoin, and his condition worsened with advanced delirium and urinary incontinence. Noticing dark-colored urine and a high titer of 1:80 porphobilinogen in urine, the diagnosis of porphyria was suspected. Due to untimely diagnosis and treatment, the patient fell into coma and died 5 days later.

According to foreign scientists, the age and gender distribution among 6 patients diagnosed with porphyria showed: 5 cases were female and 1 male; the average age of patients was 28.5 years. Cases of acute intermittent porphyria were most frequent in females between the second and fourth decade of life. The mean age of the patients was 27.6 years. The mean number of episodes was 2.83. Among 6 patients, 4 patients presented with abdominal pain, autonomic instability, psychiatric symptoms were noted in all 6 patients. Depression was found in 3 patients and delirium symptoms were observed in 2 patients. Depression and delirium are the two neuropsychiatric manifestations that most commonly accompany porphyria. Seizures were observed in 3 of the patients [120].

Watson-Schwartz tests are always positive during episodes of neuropsychiatric dysfunction, but the urine porphobilinogen concentration is 3 to 5 times the upper limit of normal. Depression is common in porphyria, but all textbooks are silent regarding the safety of taking antidepressants. There is uncertainty regarding new antidepressants for porphyria in depressed patients. Regarding the use of haloperidol and other phenothiazine-type antipsychotics, the textbooks are silent about them. Theoretically we know that drugs that metabolize "cytochrome P450" enzyme systems in the liver result in heme consumption by cytochrome P450. Which leads to a decrease in cellular heme concentration levels, and in turn a decrease in alanine synthetase concentration with an increase in the rate of heme synthesis, which can lead to increased porphobilinogen production in patients.

AFTERLIFE.

Thus, while in the first part of the monograph I used scientifically based arguments, in the second part, on the contrary, I used testimonies of people who have lived through the experience of dying. But which of these two opposites is the truth? There is an expression: "Man is the measure of all things". I think it will be most appropriate here. Each person will interpret the meaning of what is said through the prism of his emotional experience. That is what will be the truth for him.

As for the topic of the monograph, I came to the conclusion that it is impossible to die with dignity after euthanasia: the sin of this murder will lead to consequences - the soul will suffer even after death. What about the stages of existence of "life after death" described by R. Moody?

Will the souls of those "killed by mercy" be able to meet there with the "luminous being" - the embodiment of love and forgiveness?

On the other hand, maybe the suffering of these people arises for a reason. Being on the threshold between life and death, left to themselves, these people finally realize that no one can help them, they desperately turn to the medical profession to get an answer to their question, they want to die with dignity, but, in fact, they are not prepared for death. A person who finds himself in such a situation is given a great opportunity to summarize his existence, to reflect on the pictures of his life, and to understand what has become available to people who have experienced clinical death. And perhaps then they will no longer be afraid of death. Love of neighbor is something that has been revealed to many who have gone through the experience of dying. Compassionate killing cannot be a manifestation of such love. We deceive ourselves when we say "mercy killing". Lying to save the sick cannot be sweet. A lie remains a lie.

If I were asked, "Do you allow euthanasia?" *I* would say, "Under no circumstances." I think so as a doctor and as a human being.

The law should stop distinguishing between permissible and impermissible decisions to end a life based on concepts such as action-restraint from action, causing-not causing death, and intent-absence of intent to cause death.

Among the reasons why patients requested euthanasia in the Netherlands (a country where euthanasia is legalized by the state), loss of dignity ranked first, pain second, and undignified dying third.

In the Russian Federation, cases of organ harvesting for transplantation from donors with "irreversible brain death," i.e., still preserved heart function and partial brain stem function, have long been legalized. Does saving another person's life justify such sacrifices? And what would happen if euthanasia were legalized?

Circumstances that bring the life interests of the mother into conflict with the life interests of the child create a dilemma: Can a pregnancy be intentionally terminated or not? And can human life be willfully terminated or not? After all, we don't call abortion "mercy killing," do we?

Laws and the Church - their view on the problem of "medical termination of life" in L. Durov's publication "Euthanasia - easy death?".

The sociological survey of Moscow doctors opens a veil on the attitude of medical professionals to this problem. Young specialists tend to allow euthanasia more often than the category of older age group; medical professions that are directly related to saving human life - anesthesiologists, and neurologists, facing sluggish chronic diseases that cannot be treated; employees of research institutes due to research interest more often than general physicians.

Is there life after death according to the testimonies of survivors of clinical death from the book "Life After Life" by Raymond Moody, PhD.

In 30 years, the Netherlands has moved from euthanasia for the terminally ill, to euthanasia for those who are chronically ill; from euthanasia for physical illness, to euthanasia for mental illness; from euthanasia for mental illness, to euthanasia for psychological discomfort or mental suffering - and now to euthanasia simply if a person is over 70 and "tired of living." Dutch euthanasia protocols have also moved from conscious patients, rendering euthanasia with explicit consent, to subconscious patients who are unable to consent. Denial of euthanasia or assisted suicide in the Netherlands is now considered a form of discrimination against people with chronic illnesses, whether the illness may be physical or psychological, because these people will be forced to "suffer" more than those who are terminally ill. Involuntary euthanasia is now a justifiable way to appeal to the public duty of citizens and ethical positions of mercy. In the Netherlands, euthanasia has evolved from being a last resort to being one of the early manifestations of medical intervention. Belgium has followed suit [73], and disturbing evidence of euthanasia comes from Oregon, particularly with regard to the protection of depressed people and the objectivity of the process.

The United Nations found that the right to euthanasia in the Netherlands was established in violation of the Universal Declaration of Human Rights because of the danger to the individual and the threat to the integrity to life of every human being. The UN also expressed concern that the system may fail to detect and prevent situations in which people may be subjected to undue pressure to provide consent to euthanasia and may circumvent safeguards. Autonomy and choice are important values in any society, but they too are not without limitations. Our democratic society has legalized many laws that limit individual autonomy and choice so that society provides for larger communities. Legislators in some countries and jurisdictions, last year, voted against legalizing euthanasia and assisted suicide in part because of the concerns and evidence described in this review article. Those jurisdictions include France, Scotland, England, South Australia, and New Hampshire. They favored improving palliative care services and educating health care providers and the public.

Euthanasia: the practice of deliberately ending a life in order to alleviate suffering. The word "euthanasia" comes from the Greek "eu", beautiful or good+ "thanatos", death= good death. It refers to a situation where a physician contributes to the death of a patient by lethal injection who is non-viable and persistently asks the physician to euthanize him or her [79].

The Netherlands is the only country in the world where euthanasia is practiced openly. It is not specifically authorized by law, but Dutch law adopts standards of protection against physicians who must adhere to official guidelines. These guidelines are based on the voluntariness of the patient's request and relief of suffering. Euthanasia and assisted suicide are defined by the state's Euthanasia Commission. Euthanasia is the intentional termination of the life of someone other than the person concerned at his or her request. Suicide means intentionally helping a patient to terminate his or her life at his or her request. Under Dutch law, euthanasia is the termination of life by a physician at the express will of the patient. Upon request to the physician, the patient's will must be voluntary, explicit and scrutinized, the conclusion must be made more than once. Moreover, the patient's suffering must be unbearable and without any prospect of improvement. Because of the pain, a Dutch doctor can shorten a patient's life. As in other countries, this action is considered a normal medical decision to end a patient's life, not euthanasia.

Many articles have shown that HIV infection can alter the clinical course of leprosy, but very few epidemiologic and clinical data on this co-infection are found in the available literature. This literature review describes the geographic distribution and demographic characteristics in 92 HIV/ Mycobacterium leprae co-infected patients who received skilled care at the

Brazilian Leprosy Reference Center. This article describes a multivariate analysis that was used to establish the clinical features of the course of type 1 leprosy reactions. The analysis of recent referral data from the reference center showed that the number of patients with co-infection has been steadily increasing over the past years. The prevalence of leprosy was more frequent among men aged 32.3 years. Use of antiretroviral therapy was the only factor associated with type 1 leprosy response. Most patients lived in the central part of the region or in the northern part of Rio de Janeiro, Brazil. Patients with HIV and leprosy were more likely to be from regions characterized by a high density of impoverished populations.

REFERENCE LIST:

1	. Bykova C., Yudin B., Yasnaya L. What doctors think about euthanasia // Vrach. - 1994. -№ 4.- c. 48-51.

2	. Vlasov V. On the attractiveness of death and euthanasia // Physician. -1999.-№ 2.- p. 44-45.

3	. Joni E., Joe M. Joni.- Light in the East.- 1988.- 259 pp.

4	. Durnov L. Euthanasia - easy death? // Vrach.- 1998.-№ 7.- pp. 43-45.

5	. Cuse X. "No" to distinguishing between intention and foresight in medical end-of-life decisions // International Journal of Medicine.- 1998.-№ 4.- pp. 357360.

6	. Moody R. Life after life. The study of the phenomenon of continuation of life after the death of the body: Per. from English / Preface by Dr. E. Kubler-Ross.- M.: "Fizkultura i Sport", SP "Intercontact", 1990.- 92 p.

7	. A little about the past / Euthanasia - mercy killing? A. Grando - K.: 2003.- 228 p.

8	. We discuss the article by L. Durov "Euthanasia - easy death?" // Vrach. 1998.-№ 11.- p. 40-41.

9	. Popova L.M. Ethical problems arising in the diagnosis of brain death: Review // Anesthesiology and Reanimatology.- 1992.-№ 5.- pp. 69-72.

10	.USSR. Ministry of Health. Order No. 191 of 15.02.85 on the approval of the "Temporary Instruction on Death Constantation".

11	.A study of Canadian Hospice Palliative Care Volunteer's Attitudes toward physician - assisted suicide / Stephen Claxton - Oldfield, Kathryn Miller // American Journal of Hospice and Palliative Medicine. - 2015. - Vol. 32. - №3.- P. 305 - 312.

12	Burleigh M. Death and delivery: Euthanasia in Germany, 1900 - 1945 / Burleigh M., Boyd C.E.. - History: Reviews of New Books. - Taylor and Francis, 1995.

13	Defining dignity in terminally ill cancer patients: A factor - analytic approach / Thomas F., Hack Harvey Max, Chochinov Thomas [et al.] // Psycho - Oncology. - 2004. - Vol. 13. - P. 1000 - 1002.

14	Dieter Birnbacher. Euthanasia / Dieter Birnbacher // International Encyclopedia of the Social and Behavioral Sciences. - 2015. - P. 280 - 284.

15	Differences in parent-provider concordance regarding prognosis and goals of care among children with advanced cancer / Abby R. Rosenberg, Liliana Orellana, Tammy I. Kang, J. Russell Geyer, Chris Feudtner, Veronica Dussel, Joanne Wolfe // Journal of clinical oncology. - 2014. - Vol. 32. - №27,- P. 3005 - 3011.

16   Eduard Verhagen A.A. Neonatal euthanasia: Lessons from the Groningen Protocol / Eduard Verhagen A.A. // Seminars in Fetal and Neonatal Medicine. - 2014. - Vol. 19. - P. 296 - 299.

17   Emergency physicians and physician-assisted suicide, part I: A review of the physician-assisted suicide debate / John C., Moskop Kenneth V., Iserson L. // Annals of Emergency Medicine. - 2001. - Vol. 38. - P. 570 - 575.

18   .End - of - life decision making in neonates and infants: comparison of the Netherlands and Belgium / Astrid M., Vrakking Agnes, Van Der Heide Veerle [et al.] // Acta Paediatrica. - 2007. - Vol. 96. - P. 820 - 824.

19   .End - of - life decisions in individuals dying with dementia in Belgium / Kenneth Chambaere, Joachim Cohen, Lenzo Robijn MSc., S. Kathleen Bailey, Luc Deliens // Journal of the American Geriatric Society. - 2015. - Volume 63, Issue 2. - P. 290 - 296.

20   End - of - life medical decisions in France: a death certificate follow - up survey 5 years after the 2005 act of parliament on patients' rights and end of life / Sophie Pennec Alain, Monnier Silvia, Pontone Regis Aubry // BMC Palliative Care. - 2012. - Vol. 11. - P. 25 - 30.

21   European public acceptance of euthanasia: Socio-demographic and cultural factors associated with the acceptance of euthanasia in 33 European countries / Joachim Cohenlsabelle, Marcoux Johan, Bilsen Patrick [et al.] // Social Science and Medicine. - 2006. - Vol. 63. - P. 743 - 756.

22   . Euthanasia and other medical decisions concerning the end of life / P.J. van der Maas, J.J.M. van Delden, L. Hijnenborg MSc., C.W.N. Looman MSc. // The Lancet. - 1991. - Vol. 338 (8768). - P. 669 - 674.

23   Euthanasia and physician-assisted suicide: attitudes and experiences of oncology patients, oncologists, and the public / E.J. Emanuel. Emanuel, E.R. Daniels, D.L. Fairclough, B.R. Clarridge // The Lancet. - 1996. - Vol. 347 (9018). - P. 1805 - 1810.

24   Euthanasia, Physician-Assisted Suicide, and Other Medical Practices Involving the End of Life in the Netherlands, 1990 - 1995 / Paul J. van der Maas, Gerrit van der Wal, Ilinka Haverkate [et al.] // New England Journal of Medicine. - 1996. - Vol. 335. - P. 1699 - 1705.

25   French intensives do not apply American recommendations regarding decisions to forgo life - sustaining therapy / Frederic Pochard Elie, Azoulay Sylvie, Chevret Christophe [et al.] // Critical Care Medicine. - 2001. - Vol. 29. - P. 1887 - 1892.

26   J.J.M. van Delden. Euthanasia (Physician - Assisted Suicide) / J.J.M. van Delden //

Encyclopedia of Applied Ethics (Second Edition). - 2012. - P. 200 - 207.

27   Jecker N.S. Ethics and Euthanasia / N.S. Jecker // Encyclopedia of Gerontology. - 2007. - P. 522 - 525.

28   .Legalizing assisted suicide - views of physicians in Oregon / Lee M.A., Nelson H.D., Tilden V.P., Ganzini L., Schmidt T.A., Tolle S.W.. // New England Journal of Medicine. - 1996. - Vol. 334. - P. 310 - 315.

29   .Michael Wunder. Learning with History: Nazi Medical Crimes and Today's Debates on Euthanasia in Germany. - 2015. - Vol. 27. - P. 301 - 312.

30   .Mobius G. Ethical and legal questions regarding the killing of animals to avoid considerable pain and suffering / Mobius G. // Dtsch. Tierarztl Wochenschr. - 1994. - № 101 (9). - P. 372 - 376.

31   Physician-assisted suicide and euthanasia in Washington State: patient requests and physician responses / Black A.L., Wallace J.I., Starks H.E., Pearlman R.A. // JAMA. - 1996. - Vol. 275. - P. 919 - 925.

32   Position paper on euthanasia. Utrecht, the Netherlands: Royal Dutch Medical Association, 1995.

33   Trends in end - of -life practices before the enactment of the euthanasia law in the Netherlands from 1990 to 2010: a repeated cross - sectional survey / Bregje D., Onwuteaka - Philipsen Arianne, Brinkman - Stoppelenburg Corine [et al.]. - The Lancet. - 2012. - Vol. 380. - P. 908 - 915.

34   .Van der Wal G., van der Maas P.J.. Euthanasie en andere medische beslissingen rond het levenseinde. The Hague, the Netherlands: Staatsuitgeverij, 1996.

35   .Woodruff R. Dutch experience of euthanasia / Woodruff R. // The Lancet. - 2001. - Vol. 358. - P. 667 - 668.

36   Alaberdeeva Г.Р. Euthanasia as a medical and social problem / G.R. Alaberdeeva // Bulletin of Saratov State Technical University. - 2007. - Issue 3. - Vol. 1.- P. 1- 17.

37   Aliev T.T. Euthanasia in Russia: the human right to its realization // Modern Law. - 2008. - № 4. - C. 48.

38   .Wagatsuma S., Ariizumi T. Civil Law of Japan. - M., 1993. - C. 12.

39   Dovbush A. The right to a dignified death / A. Dovbush // Law of Ukraine. - 2002. - № 10. - C. 124.

40   Life of Lycurgus// Plutarch. Selected hagiographies: V2 - х т.-M., 1986. -T.1.-C. 108.

41   Zilber A.P. Treatise on Euthanasia. - Petrozavodsk: PetrSU, 1998. - C. 344 - 345.

42   Ivanyushkin A.Ya. Professional ethics in medicine / A.Ya. Ivanyushkin. - M.: Medicine, 1990. - 130 c.

43   Ivchenko, I. A. Euthanasia as an expression of free will and the right to death (historical and philosophical analysis) / I. A. Ivchenko // Izvestia of the Russian State Pedagogical University named after A. I. Herzen. - 2009. - Issue № 107. - C. 20 - 27.

44   Koni A.F. Koni's Collected Works in 8 volumes. - M.: Yuridicheskaya Literatura, 1996. - T. 4. Suicide in law and life. - 480 c.

45   .Mercer F.W. Australia hands out euthanasia kits [Electronic resource].   - Mode   access: http://news .bbc.co.uk/hi/russian/life/newsid 2204000/2204836. stm

46   Olkhovik L.A. Legal regulation of euthanasia: domestic and foreign opit / L.A. Olkhovik // South Ukrainian legal bulletin. - 2012. - №3.- C. 59 - 62.

47   Monuments of Roman law. Laws of XII tables. Institutions of Gaius and Digests of Justinian. -M., 1997. - C. 6.

48   Romanovsky G.B. Euthanasia: annals of history // Medical Law. - 2007. - № 3 (19). - C. 17.

49   .Simonov A. Euthanasia: to die cannot live // Yuridicheskiy Mir. - 2005. - №3.-C. 34-42.

50   .Sivryuk K. Euthanasia for minors in the context of the right to life / K. Sivryuk // Family and Law: national and international aspects: second legal readings, December 11, 2014. - Kharkiv, 2014.

51   Slavkina N.A. Euthanasia: for and against (legal aspects) // Modern Problems of Law and State. - M., 1990. - C. 156 - 157.

52   Stefanchuk R.A. Returning to the question of legalization of euthanasia in CIS countries // State and Law. - 2008. - № 5.- C. 76.

53   Tsymbaliuk V. Criminal liability of medical workers for crimes against human life and health: directions of reforming the legislation / V. Tsymbaliuk // Historico-legal chasopis. - Lutsk, 2014. - №2 (4). - C. 111 - 115.

54   Chernysheva, Yu.A. Legal regulation of euthanasia in foreign countries // Law and Law. - 2008. - №6. - C. 109.

55   Shevchuk S.S. Problems of legal regulation of relations on rendering medical services.

- Stavropol: "Stavropolservice - school", 2007. - 332 c.

56	.Deliens L, van der Wal G. The euthanasia law in Belgium and the Netherlands. Lancet. 2003;362:1239-40.

57	.Watson R. Luxembourg is to allow euthanasia. BMJ. 2009;338:b1248.

58	.Steinbrook R. Physician-assisted death-from Oregon to Washington State. N Engl J Med. 2008;359:2513-15.

59	.Hurst S, Mauron A. Assisted suicide and euthanasia in Switzerland: allowing a role for non-physicians. BMJ.2003;326:271-3.

60	. Smets T, Bilsen J, Cohen J, Rurup ML, De Keyser E, Deliens L. The medical practice of euthanasia in Belgium and the Netherlands: legal notification, control and evaluation procedures. Health Policy. 2009;90:181- 7.

61	. Caplan AL, Snyder L, Faber-Langendoen K. The role of guidelines in the practice of physician-assisted suicide. University of Pennsylvania Center for Bioethics Assisted Suicide Consensus Panel. Ann Intern Med.2000;132:476-81.

62	.Van der Heide A, Onwuteaka-Philipsen BD, Rurup ML, et al. End-of-life practices in the Netherlands under the *Euthanasia Act*. N Engl J Med. 2007;356:1957-65. 8. Van den Block L, Deschepper R, Bilsen J, Bossuyt N, Van Casteren V, Deliens L. Euthanasia and other end-of-life decisions and care provided in the final three months of life: nationwide retrospective study in Belgium. BMJ.2009;339:b2772.

63	. Van den Block L, Deschepper R, Bilsen J, Bossuyt N, Van Casteren V, Deliens L. Euthanasia and other end-of-life decisions: a mortality follow-up study in Belgium. BMC Public Health. 2009; 9:79.

64	.Chambaere K, Bilsen J, Cohen J, Onwuteaka-Philipsen BD, Mortier F, Deliens L. Physician-assisted deaths under the euthanasia law in Belgium: a population-based survey. CMAJ. 2010;182:895-901.

65	.Smets T, Bilsen J, Cohen J, Rurup ML, Mortier F, Deliens L. Reporting of euthanasia in medical practice in Flanders, Belgium: cross sectional analysis of reported and unreported cases. BMJ. 2010;341:c5174.

66	.Inghelbrecht E, Bilsen J, Mortier F, Deliens L. The role of nurses in physician-assisted deaths in Belgium.CMAJ. 2010;182:905-10.

67	.Chochinov HM, Wilson KG, Enns M, et al. Desire for death in the terminally ill. Am J Psychiatry.1995;152:1185-91.

68   .Emanuel EJ, Fairclough DL, Emanuel LL. Attitudes and desires related to euthanasia and physician-assisted suicide among terminally ill patients and their caregivers. JAMA. 2000;284:2460-8.

69   .Breitbart W, Rosenfeld B, Pessin H, et al. Depression, hopelessness, and desire for hastened death in terminally ill patients with cancer. JAMA. 2000;284:2907-11.

70   .Smith SW. Evidence for the practical slippery slope in the debate on physician assisted suicide and euthanasia.Med Law Review. 2005;13:17-44.

71   . Sheldon T. Dutch GP found guilty of murder faces no penalty. BMJ. 2001;322:509.

72   Bilsen J, Cohen J, Chambaere K, et al. Medical end-of-life practices under the euthanasia law in Belgium. N Engl J Med. 2009;361:1119-21.

73   . Smets T, Bilsen J, Cohen J, Rurup ML, Deliens L. Legal euthanasia in Belgium: characteristics of all reported euthanasia cases. Med Care. 2010;48:187-92.

74   .Verhagen AA, Sol JJ, Brouwer OF, Sauer PJ. Deliberate termination of life in newborns in the Netherlands; review of all 22 reported cases between 1997 and 2004 Ned Tijdschr Geneeskd. 2005;149:183-8.

75   .Sheldon T. Dutch law leads to confusion over when to use life ending treatment in suffering newborns. BMJ.2009;339:b5474.

76   .Burgermeister J. Doctor reignites euthanasia row in Belgium after mercy killing. BMJ. 2006;332:382.

77   .Cohen-Almagor R. Belgian euthanasia law: a critical analysis. J Med Ethics. 2009;35:436-9.

78   . Wilson K, Chochinov HM, McPherson CJ, et al. Desire for euthanasia or physician-assisted   suicide   in palliative cancer care. Health Psychol. 2007;26:314-23.

79   .Bernheim J, Deschepper R, Distelmans W, Mullie A, Bilsen J, Deliens L. Development of palliative care and legalization of euthanasia: antagonism or synergy? BMJ. 2008;336:864-7.

80   .George RJD, Finlay IG, Jeffrey D. Legalized euthanasia will violate the rights of vulnerable patients. BMJ.2005;331:684-5.

81   .Euthanasia [letter] Lancet. 1991;338:1150.

82   .Zylicz Z. Hospice in Holland: the story behind the blank spot. Am J Hosp Palliat Care. 1993;10:30-4.

83   .United Kingdom . Human Rights Act 1998. London, U.K.: United Kingdom; 1998. Schedule 1, Article 2.1. [Available online at:www.legislation.gov.uk/ukpga/1998/42/schedule/1 ; cited February 17, 2011].

84   .Oregon Department of Human Services (DHS), Office of Disease Prevention and Epidemiology . *Sixth Annual Report on Oregon 's* Death with Dignity Act. Portland, OR: dhs; 2004. [Available online at:www.oregon.gov/DHS/ph/pas/docs/year6.pdf ; cited February 17, 2011]

85   .Finlay IG, George R. Legal physician-assisted suicide in Oregon and the Netherlands: evidence concerning the impact on patients in vulnerable groups; another perspective on Oregon's data. J Med Ethics. 2010.

86   .Portenoy RK, Coyle N, Kash KM, et al. Determinants of the willingness to endorse assisted suicide: a survey of physicians, nurses, and social workers. Psychosomatics. 1997;38:277-87.

87   .Zylicz B. Palliative care and euthanasia in the Netherlands: observations of a Dutch physician. In: Foley KM, Hendin H, editors. The Case Against Assisted Suicide: For the Right to End-of-Life Care. Baltimore, MD: Johns Hopkins University Press; 2002.

88   .Emanuel EJ. Depression, euthanasia, and improving end-of-life care. J Clin Oncol. 2005;23:6456-8.

89   .Chochinov HM, Hack T, Hassard T, Kristjanson LJ, McClement S, Harlos M. Dignity therapy: a novel psychotherapeutic intervention for patients near the end of life. J Clin Oncol. 2005;23:5520-5.

90   .Morgado MG, Barcellos C, Pina MF, et al. Human immunodeficiency virus/acquired immunodeficiency syndrome and tropical diseases: a Brazilian perspective. Mem Inst Oswaldo Cruz 2000;95(Suppl 1):145- 51.CrossRefMedlineWeb of ScienceGoogle Scholar

91   .Orsini M, Canela JR, Disch J, et al. High frequency of asymptomatic Leishmania spp. infection among HIV-infected patients living in endemic areas for visceral leishmaniasis in Brazil. Trans R Soc Trop Med Hyg 2012;106:283-8.doi:10.1016/j.trstmh.2012.01.008.

92   .Co-infection: new battlegrounds in HIV/AIDS. Lancet Infect Dis 2013;13:559

93   .Pavie J, De Castro N, Molina JM, et al. Severe peripheral neuropathy following HAART initiation in an HIV-infected patient with leprosy. J Int Assoc Physicians AIDS Care (Chic) 2010;9:232- 5. doi: 10.1177/1545109710373829.

1.   .Sarno EN, Illarramendi X, Nery JA, et al. HIV-M. leprae interaction: can HAART modify the course of leprosy? leprae interaction: can HAART modify the course of leprosy? Public Health Rep 2008;123:206-12. MedlineWeb of ScienceGoogle Scholar

95.   Talhari C, Mira MT, Massone C, et al. Leprosy and HIV coinfection: a clinical, pathological, immunological, and therapeutic study of a cohort from a Brazilian referral center for infectious diseases. J Infect Dis 2010;202:345- 54.

96.   Couppie P, Domergue V, Clyti E, et al. Increased incidence of leprosy following HAART initiation: a manifestation of the immune reconstitution disease. AIDS2009;23:1599-600. doi:10.1097/QAD.0b013e32832bb5b7.

97.   WHO. Geneva: World Health Organization; 2012. Weekly Epidemiologic Record: Global leprosy situation. http://www.who.int/wer/2012/wer8734.pdf [accessed August 13, 2013].

98.   Jopling WH McDougall AC. Leprosy Reactions. In: Jopling WH, McDougall AC (eds). Handbook of Leprosy. 5th th ed. New Delhi: 82, CBS Publishers and Distributors Pvt. Ltd. Ltd.; 1996. p. 82-91.

99.   Sharma VK, Malhotra AK. Leprosy: Classification and clinical aspects. In: Valia RG, Valia AR, editors. IADVL Textbook of dermatology. 3rd rd ed. Mumbai: Bhalani Publishing House; 2008. p. 2032.

100.   Sharma VK, Malhotra AK. Leprosy: Classification and clinical aspects. In: Valia RG, Valia AR, editors. IADVL Textbook of dermatology. 3rd rd ed. Mumbai: Bhalani Publishing House; 2008. p. 2032-69.

101.   Ustianowski AP, Lawn SD, Lockwood DN. Interactions between HIV infection and leprosy: A paradox. Lancet Infect Dis 2006;6:350-60.

102.   Sanghi S, Grewal RS, Vasudevan B, Lodha N. Immune reconstitution inflammatory syndrome in leprosy. Indian J Lepr 2011;83:61-70.

103.   Nigam P, Goyal BM, Mishra DN, Samuel KC. Reaction in leprosy complicated by filariasis. Lepr India 1977;49:344-8.

104.   Vinay K, Smita J, Nikhil G, Neeta G. Human immunodeficiency virus and leprosy co-infection in Pune, India. J Clin Microbiol 2009;47:2998-9.

105.   Pai VV, Tayshetye PU, Ganapati R. Observations in 11 patients with leprosy and humanimmunodeficiency virus co-association. Indian J Dermatol Venereol Leprol 2011;77:714-6.

106. Sharma NL, Mahajan VK, Sharma VC, Sarin S, Sharma RC. Erythema nodosum leprosum and HIV infection: A therapeutic experience. Int J Lepr Other Mycobact Dis 2005;73:189-93.

107. Sachdeva S, Amin SS, Qaisar S. Type 2 lepra reaction with HIV1 coinfection: A case report with interesting management implications. Indian J Lepr 2011;83:103-6.

108. Abdul Rahman R, Hwen-Yee C, Noordin R. Pan LF-ELISA using BmR1 and BmSXP recombinant antigens for detection of lymphatic filariasis. Filaria J 2007;6:10.

109. Ackner B, Cooper JE, Gray CH, et al. Acute porphyria-a neuropsychiatric and biochemical study. J Psychosom Res. 962;6:1-24.

110. Goldberg A. Acute intermittent porphyria: A study of 50 cases. Q J Med. 1959;28:183-209.

111. Tishler PV, Woodward B, O'Connor J, et al. High prevalence of intermittent acute porphyria in a psychiatric patient population. Am J Psychiatry. 1985;142:1320-36.

112. Paramala SJ, Malhotra S. Varied psychiatric manifestations of acute intermittent porphyria. Biol Psychiatry.1994;136:744-7.

113. Burgovne K, Swartz R, Ananth J. Porphyria: Reexamination of psychiatric implications. Psychother Psychosom.1995;64:121-30.

114. Sugimara K. Acute intermittent porphyria. Nippon Rinsho. 1995;53:1418-21.

115. Bandr ES, Sanchez MP, Reynaog P. Acute intermittent porphyria at the hospital Arzobispo Loay-za of Lima (1983-1994)-A report of 14 cases. Rev Gastroenterology Peru. 1994;14:209-14.

116. Bylesjo I, Forsgren L, Lithner F, et al. Epidemiology and clinical characteristics of seizures in patients with acute intermittent porphyria. Epilepsia. 1996;37:230-5.

117. Jeans JB, Savik K, Gross CR, et al. Mortality in patients with acute intermittent porphyria requiring hospitalization: A United States Case Series. Am J Med Genet. 1996;65:269-73.

118. Reio LQ, Wetterberg L. False porphobilinogen reactions in the urine of mental patients. JAMA.1969;207:148-50.

119. Crimlisk HL. The little imitator-Porphyria: A neuro-psychiatric disorder. J Neurol Neurosurg Psychiatry. 1997;62:319-28.

120. Chatterjee MN, Rana S. Textbook of medical biochemistry. New Delhi: Jaypee Brothers; 1993. Porphyrias and porphyrinurias; pp. 300-15.

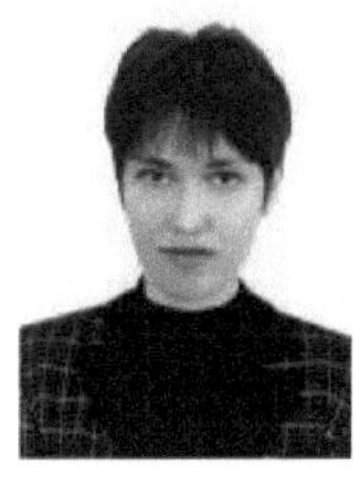**Grigorenko Lyubov Viktorovna**, Candidate of Medical Sciences, Associate Professor of the Department of Hygiene and Ecology "Dnepropetrovsk Medical Academy of MHI", doctoral student. Second higher education in the direction of training 6.020303 "Specialist in Philology. Translator of the English language". Conducts practical classes and consultations, gives lectures on the subject: "General hygiene and ecology" for English-speaking foreign students and students of medical faculties of VI courses in the specialty: "Medicine".

Author of 130 publications: 79 scientific and 51 educational and methodological, including 17 in fakh publications. After defending her PhD thesis, she published 102 scientific articles: 59 - in scientific journals and 43 educational-methodical, including 14 works in fakh publications, 10 - foreign articles, 4 - in international scientometric journals; 10 teaching aids for English-speaking students; 6 author's certificates.

Member of the Federation of the National Team of Scientists of the IASHE international project (in London). Three times she was awarded a bronze medal for the best publication in English as a prize-winner of the I, II and III stages of competitions in the branch "Medicine and Pharmacy, Biology, Veterinary Medicine and Agriculture", section: "Hygiene".

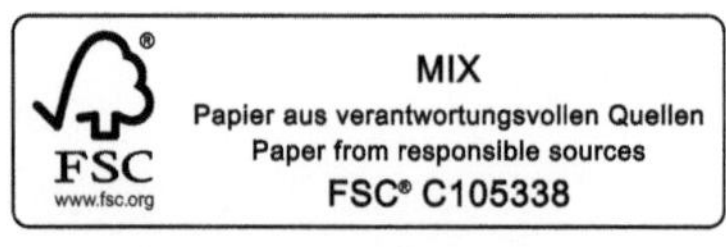

Printed by Books on Demand GmbH, Norderstedt / Germany